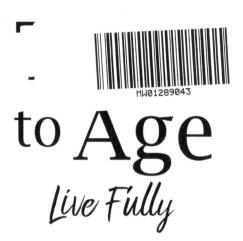

to **Age**

Live Fully

Joni Grant

outskirts
press

Outskirts Press, Inc.
http://www.outskirtspress.com

ISBN: 978-1-9772-4613-4

Library of Congress Control Number: 2021917109

Cover Photo © 2021 www.gettyimages.com. All rights reserved - used with
permission.

Outskirts Press and the "OP" logo are trademarks belonging to Outskirts
Press, Inc.

PRINTED IN THE UNITED STATES OF AMERICA

This book is dedicated to my clients who inspire me every day. To Justin and Amanda who took a chance and hired a sixty-three-year-old personal trainer when they opened their Anytime Fitness. To my beautiful daughter who seems to believe that I can do just about anything! And nothing great is ever accomplished without the love and support of friends. I am thankful for every one of them who has cheered me on to this final finished product.

Disclaimer

The author strongly recommends that you consult with your physician before beginning any exercise program. You should be in good physical condition and be able to participate in the exercise. The author is not a licensed healthcare care provider and represents that they have no expertise in diagnosing, examining, or treating medical conditions of any kind, or in determining the effect of any specific exercise on a medical condition. You should understand that when participating in any exercise or exercise program, there is the possibility of physical injury. If you engage in this exercise or exercise program, you agree that you do so at your own risk, are voluntarily participating in these activities, assume all risk of injury to yourself, and agree to release and discharge the author from any and all claims or causes of action, known or unknown, arising out of the contents of this book.

Table of Contents

Introduction

"We do not stop exercising because we grow old. We grow old because we stop exercising."

—Dr. Kenneth Cooper

You get to decide how you age. Is that news to you? Do you think aging is a natural process that we all go through? Would you believe me if I told you there is nothing "natural" about the way we age in America? We are not built to spend the last thirty years of our life on the couch. Movement is as important to you now as it was when you were a ten-year-old. To age well, you have to keep moving. But movement is only the beginning of the story.

I hope you are curious enough to read on, because your quality of life, for the last third of your life, will be determined by your belief in what I am about to share with you. More importantly, I want you to act on that belief. Reading this book does nothing for you unless you take action. And that action can change your life! I have tried to simplify complex topics. I want this book to be a quick, easy read, and I hope the end of this book is indeed a new beginning for you. Aging can be challenging, and this book is one of the many tools you can use to be a successful, active ager.

But first, let me introduce myself. I am currently a personal trainer, but I previously spent twenty-five years behind a desk. I have been overweight for a good portion of my life and am an ex-smoker. As far as exercise, I would jump into a program and then quit. I probably did that fifty times in my life. I am not the profile of a person who should be writing about fitness. But here I am. I am like many other people my age, which at this writing is sixty-five. And I'm here to tell you that getting old is not for the faint of heart. Aging isn't fun. It's hard, and sometimes it's downright depressing. Some days it feels like I take one step forward and two steps backward. That said, working out and building strength and balance at least lets me make this journey on my terms. And that feeling, that hope, is what I want for you. I want you to travel down this road called aging on your terms.

You may be getting older and finding your joints are getting stiff. Getting out of a chair takes more effort as each year passes. You may have started rolling yourself out of your chair by throwing your body weight forward to give yourself enough momentum to stand up. Do you remember the last time you were able to get down on the floor and back up again with any kind of strength or grace? Do you avoid getting down on the floor with grandkids because you can't get up and you refuse to ask for help? Or, do you see the time approaching when you can't get up off the floor, and you're just resigned to it? It's just one more thing that you give up as you age.

Maybe you've given up hope, and you believe the future is simply a downhill trip to the end of your life. Here's the truth. Regardless of what we do, we're all on a downhill journey to the end of our lives. This book is about your quality of life as you approach the end of life.

I am not a nutritionist and will not be covering nutrition except to tell you that you probably are not getting enough protein. This book is not about weight loss. It's about getting started working out now! I have a bad knee and just recovered from two surgeries for breast cancer. I have started my fitness program over due to injury or illness more than once and will probably have to start over many more times. Fitness for an active ager isn't a straight line. You can expect hills, gullies, and U-turns in your journey. The good news is that the only way you can go wrong is not getting back to the program as soon as you can.

You work out for your health and longevity. You wouldn't wait to take aspirin until the headache was gone, would you? Don't allow physical appearance or lack of experience to stop you from getting started or restarted. You will find that starting wherever you are provides results and sets an example for others. Be brave; read on and give it a try.

My whole journey started with "twenty seconds of courage," a phrase I became familiar with in 2016 at Camp Nerd Fitness, created by Steve Kamb. It was a camp built around health and fitness, and it's where I truly learned just how much you could accomplish if you simply take those precious twenty seconds to try something new. For many of us, starting a fitness journey at age fifty, sixty, or seventy is a challenge that requires that magical twenty seconds of courage to begin.

I am going to throw out one more term you need to know: "compression of morbidity." It sounds like a complex term, but it simply means reducing how much time you spend sick or disabled. That's precisely what we all want. We want to be healthy, independent, and active for as long as possible, and we want to reduce the amount of time we are disabled or ill. *Train to Age* is all about extending the quality of your life. My goal is to be as healthy and fit for as long as I can. I hope those are your goals too. Read on, and you'll find that you do have some choice in how you age.

In this book, I am going to introduce you to some of my clients at the gym. You'll meet Carol, Lynn,

Chuck, Jan, and John. They all have their own stories, but they are much like many of you. The youngest is sixty-three, and the oldest is seventy-six. They started at the gym for various reasons at different ages. I hope their stories will inspire you to give *Train to Age* a try.

You'll also learn about many of the myths that come with aging and ageism. Maybe what you think you know about aging is just a myth someone else made up a long time ago. If you feel you're too old to start something new, you're wrong. If you're female and you didn't get much past the treadmill, there is a whole new world out there to explore. If you believe the only way to get your heart rate up is to run or jump on a treadmill or elliptical, that isn't true, and you will find you have many options. Don't be surprised if you find you enjoy strength training.

Read this book, and you'll learn how to build muscle, strengthen your bones, and become more stable and less affected by declining balance. You have to keep moving, and you'll understand why. And as an additional reward, you'll know how to reap benefits for both your heart and brain health.

There is no lack of new research on aging. I wanted to keep this book's focus on the impact of exercise, specifically resistance training and cardio, and I wanted the material to be easy to read and understand. I hope I accomplished that feat. If you want to learn more, google "resistance training and aging," and you'll find plenty of resource material.

If you're suffering from a serious injury or illness, you may need a more targeted training program than this book will provide. If you are at high risk for a bone fracture, don't exercise without checking in with your doctor. If you're frail, at increased risk for a fall, or have any other issue that would make exercise dangerous, then follow your doctor's recommendations for training.

This book is for the average person between forty and eighty. You're in decent health but find yourself getting slower, weaker, and less stable. You may have never worked out, or you've stopped because you don't see the point anymore. Or maybe you're a runner or tennis player who is watching your muscle melt away regardless of the miles you run or matches you play.

You may have arthritic knees, a bad shoulder, or one of many other issues we discover as we age. That doesn't mean you have to give up getting stronger. It just means you might have to do it a little differently.

Also, for discussions around muscle loss, the percentages I use are middle of the road. The numbers for the rate of muscle loss vary wildly, so I am on the low side. Look in the mirror. If your arms and legs have become thin and without definition, then the percentage doesn't really matter. How strong you are *does* matter.

Don't know where to start with a fitness program? I am going to give you many different options for how and where to train. Even if you have no experience working out, you can do this. By the way, if you've purchased this book for your parents, don't fool yourself. The same decline you see in your parents will happen to you. You may not believe it now, but we all get old. This book is for you too. The earlier you start, the smoother the road to old age will be.

So, regardless of who you are, let's get started on this life-changing journey.

Joni

CHAPTER 1

Beginnings

"We don't see things as they are; we see
them as we are."

—Anais Nin

I THOUGHT GETTING older was a fast slide downhill. You know the adage, "It's all downhill from here."
When I was thirty, forty was over the hill. And now,
twenty-five years past forty, I realize that when you're
forty, you're still a puppy. There are as many options
for being fit and healthy at sixty-five as there were at
forty. But at forty, I knew none of this. At forty, I thought
aging meant you lost muscle, your balance was awful, you got thick around your middle, and eventually,
you needed some kind of care to get by. That path
was the one my family traveled, and I thought, except
for a lucky few, this was the path we all walked. I

continued to hold that belief until I was the ripe old age of fifty-eight.

My mom suffered five heart attacks, the first when she was fifty. She also had COPD. My dad had a major stroke at thirty and was left paralyzed on his right side. My life experience didn't lead me to believe that I had any options for how I aged. By the time I was in my mid-fifties, I was overweight, out of shape, and had asthma from smoking. I was sure that my family's history of heart attacks and stroke would eventually catch up with me. The variable wasn't *if* but *when* it would happen. And I knew there was nothing I could do about it.

I am going to take you down a side street now, so please bear with me. In 2012, I went on a cattle drive in Wyoming. It was on my bucket list, and I was excited to check it off. I lost a lot of weight before the trip, and I was feeling pretty spunky.

We "dudes" from the city got to ride along with real cowboys moving cattle up toward the mountains for the summer. We rode beside ranch families and provided extra bodies to help keep the herds moving in the right direction. I'm not sure how useful we were, but it was fun.

What struck me were the multi-generational ranch families. Folks were riding in their seventies and eighties. They were hopping on and off horses and were faster and stronger than I have ever been at any age. This was the first time I had considered that we all didn't age at the same rate. That vacation was one of those rare moments when a tiny lightbulb goes off in the corner of your mind. It's not very bright, but you get this little glimpse of truth. I began thinking that what I knew about aging wasn't the whole story. Maybe I wasn't doomed. Could my future hold more than a downhill slide to a nursing home?

After that, not a lot changed in my life, but there was now the opportunity for change. My eyes weren't open, but I was at least getting one eyelid up on occasion. I tried playing in a pickleball league, but I faceplanted hard on a concrete court and decided that pickleball wasn't for me. I hated running and was terrified of the gym because I didn't know how to do anything but jump on a treadmill or rower. And the treadmill is my definition of hell.

About three years later, when I was almost sixty, a friend invited me to a CrossFit Box for a workout. I thought, why not? How hard can it be? I got on the rower and was deemed fit enough to join in the workout. I hung from bars, sprawled over boxes, and was generally miserable until the owner showed me how to deadlift. In that moment, I fell in love. No, not with the owner—with deadlifting.

I can tell you that what drew me in was the feeling of strength and power. These were things I hadn't felt in a very long time. Of course, I went back a second time. My second visit didn't go so well, and I decided that CrossFit wasn't for me, but picking up heavy things was!

I couldn't even tell the first couple of trainers I interviewed what I wanted to learn. Did I want to learn powerlifting? Did I want to learn weightlifting? I didn't know, so I went where everybody goes for information. I went to Google. Google led me to YouTube. YouTube got me to Women's Masters Powerlifting, and I knew I had found my nirvana. These women looked like me. They had gray hair like me. Many were round like me, and they were deadlifting, benching, and squatting at a championship level. Now that I had the words, off I went again to find a trainer. I finally found one willing to take on this weird, almost sixty-year-old woman who wanted to pick up heavy things and couldn't explain any more than that. He taught me how to train in a gym and gave me the basics of powerlifting.

By the following August, I was ready to compete in a small bench and deadlift competition at the Illinois State Fair. I was beyond terrified. Deep down in my bones, I knew that everyone was laughing at the old lady trying to deadlift. But they didn't laugh. I hit my goal of 220 pounds and got to talk to folks all day about the benefits of strength training. Some good friends came to watch, and it was a terrifying but fantastic experience.

By the end of the following year, I had two more full meets under my belt. I had lost a ton of weight, and I felt better than I ever had. I learned how to use barbells, dumbbells, kettlebells, and plate-loaded machines. I was taught how to use cables and what exercises work which muscles, and why I was doing them. I soaked the information up like a sponge. It was as if I had stepped into a whole new world that I didn't know existed. Although this makes a nice story, it was not a pretty picture. I was close to sixty, overweight, clumsy, and enamored with resistance training.

If you feel I'm not getting to the point, please bear with me. The first part of this story is important because it leads me to the place where I am now. No one ever told me that resistance training would be good for my health. I was unaware that along with increased strength, there were significant benefits for my brain and heart. I learned that strength training would improve my ability to keep my balance, as it would make me more stable. I discovered all of this after I started lifting. And I learned it by experimenting with my own body.

But here comes the part of the story you need to hear. I gained lots of strength in the process of learning to lift. That was awesome. But my blood pressure returning to a normal range was even more awesome. The fact that my balance greatly improved was another plus. I did not expect to feel healthy and strong at sixty-one, after feeling I was going downhill fast at fifty-five. That very long hill I had been sliding down since forty took a steep uphill turn, and I loved the ride.

We are all told we need to "exercise," whatever that means. I have been pointed to many treadmills by well-meaning trainers. Some attempted to murder me with cardio circuits. I purchased every DVD made, trying to get "fit." I kicked, punched, stepped, danced, and did power yoga, whatever that is. The focus for me had constantly been losing weight. That number on the scale would be my guiding star to the world of the fit and healthy. I was so wrong.

And, as we age, the answer to health and fitness becomes much more challenging. Arthritic knees and shoulders make us move a little slower in the morning. We know we must keep moving, but some days it can be downright unpleasant. You may be dealing with pills for blood pressure, cholesterol, or heart disease. Everybody has an opinion on what you should and shouldn't do as you age, including your children, doctors, and friends.

Your family history has given you a glimpse into how you might age, and if it's an awesome picture, that's great. But what if it's not? Are you doomed to die young or to spend your last years infirm and under care? Are you aware you have choices?

I didn't know I had choices. Why had no one told me anything about the benefits of resistance training? Do doctors not understand that a progressive training program has many, many benefits? Is the issue that we're seen as too fragile to do resistance training? Or maybe it's just easier to write a prescription than assume we will do what we need to do to improve our health. Could it be that we're not asking the right questions?

Many of us don't have outstanding track records at self-care. Perhaps it's up to us to take action when the doctor tells us to "get some exercise." I had one doctor who cheered me on, and one that, in so many words, told me to act my age, whatever that means. And I have a new one. I don't believe we've figured each other out yet, but she did send me for a DEXA scan. And yes, after almost seven years of resistance training, I have great bones.

Doctors tell us to do many things to stay healthy and then hand us a pill when we fail to comply. And that's on us. But now, there's a lot more at stake. After a few years of seeing my health improve, I started researching the benefits of resistance training, and I was amazed at what I discovered. This research didn't take long, and I found that there is a massive volume of information at our fingertips.

What I'm going to talk about isn't new science, and it isn't magic. It involves hard work and commitment. And if I am going to be honest, ten years ago, if someone told me what I'm going to tell you, I would have laughed in their face. After a lifetime of being pointed toward the treadmill, elliptical, and cardio workouts of all kinds, there was no reason for me to believe that a resistance training program combined with aerobic training could give me the benefits that would slow down this decline into old age. I figured at some point frailty was just something that happened to everyone, and it would happen to me, so why bother.

I didn't even know what the words strength or resistance training meant, and I would never have considered going into a weight room and touching anything, including a barbell or a kettlebell. But once I did, it was on! I backed into the information I will share with you by finding something I loved and moving forward from there. I want you to have your journey of discovering what you love and enjoying the benefits that come with it.

In the beginning, I got lots of warnings from well-meaning friends. I shouldn't pick up anything heavy because I'll get hurt. Weights will make me look like a man. No man wants a woman who is stronger than he is. All you need to do is walk every day. Don't ever pick up more than ten pounds. You're too old to be doing what you're doing. I even got that last one from a doctor. These comments are why there is a chapter on myths and ageism.

I want to be clear. I'm not suggesting you walk into the nearest gym and pick up 200 pounds. The tricky thing about older adults is we all have our worn-out parts and health histories. You should work out with your doctor's blessing and within your abilities. I train active agers from forty to eighty-plus, and they are all very different individuals. The term "active ager" refers to seniors and boomers and any other word that defines a specific generation, so you'll see it used frequently.

What is the same is that you can train, and you can improve physically. You can rebuild muscle and increase strength. Leg strength can provide stability, so you're less affected by failing balance. And you can increase the muscle fiber that lets you move faster, so you can catch yourself if you lose your balance. You won't be competing with anyone but yourself. Your focus and job will be to add quality to your life. That means living independently for as long as you can, moving well, and doing the things in life that give you pleasure. In other words, to live fully.

There are many different tools for resistance training. Moving your body weight is a great place to start, and you can move on from there. You have to find the tools that you will enjoy and keep using. And you'll need a trainer, class, group, or program to get you moving in the right direction.

What is the right direction? That's entirely up to you. We all have different expectations for our retirement years. Do you want to travel, bike, and hike across the world? Or do you plan on helping to raise your grandchildren? Chasing little ones requires energy, strength, and balance.

Maybe you plan to take up hiking or traveling the US in a motorhome. For all your dreams, you want to stay healthy and independent for as long as possible.

Whatever your retirement goals, you'll need strength, stability, strong bones, and a healthy heart and brain to achieve them.

Maybe the fact that you're struggling to get out of a chair is scaring you to death. Or you may have taken a fall, and you've suddenly realized that you just don't have the balance you had a few years ago. For me, things that had been easy were getting harder, and not only was that frustrating, but being single made it even more worrisome. I was in a desk job for most of my career and wasn't active, so I started training from ground zero. The only thing that kept me going was that I was willing to do the work because I enjoyed it. You will start from wherever you are physically and move forward from there. If you need to start in a chair class, then that's where you should start.

I will say this many times in this book. What will keep you working out and moving forward is finding fitness activities that you enjoy. There are millions of choices for both resistance training and cardio. Don't waste your time dragging yourself to a workout you hate. If you hate it, there won't be any benefits, because eventually you'll quit. Find things you can't wait to repeat because they were so much fun!

And folks, this is not about losing weight. Weight loss is a whole different subject. If you've been on the treadmill for the last thirty years thinking that you can just walk off that weight, and it hasn't happened, get off right now. Cardio will be a portion of your program, but don't put off the resistance training until you are at some magical weight. And if you need a little motivation, muscle burns more calories than fat and takes up less space per pound. With resistance training, you will build muscle and lose inches.

Powerlifting took my life in a new direction. I very much wanted to share what I'd learned, so I got my personal training certification, moved closer to my daughter's family, and began working as a trainer. Having a personal training certification doesn't make you a good trainer, but it does give you a place to start.

I worked part-time in a gym and taught a resistance training class at a local senior center. That class was where I began working more exclusively with active agers. It was clear that no one had emphasized resistance training as integral to a healthy lifestyle. I felt like I was opening a door and shining a light down a hallway that no one knew was there. I said over and over, "Yes, you can feel better, and you can be strong." And they were beginning to believe me. I was changing lives. These weren't significant changes, but they were the kind that made lives just a little better. That made me very happy, and as challenging as starting over proved to be, I knew it was worth it.

I'm now working at a brand-new Anytime Fitness, and I love the opportunity to work with many different active agers. I have people who train strength, take classes, learn to deadlift, and use all the various equipment available. I have worked hard to help my clients understand the benefits of resistance training and to believe that they can attain them.

"Belief" is an important word. If you don't think you can, you won't. I want you to believe you can. I want you to have the strength to chase your dreams regardless of your age, and I want to give you the tools you need to do that. I want you to age well and live fully. We don't know how long this ride may last, but there is no reason to turn in our train ticket before we've made it to the end of the line.

So let's start by taking a look at what happens to our bodies as we age. It's not a pretty picture, but understanding the process begins our understanding of slowing it down. The sooner you start training to age, the sooner you can impact your future!

CHAPTER 2

Compliant Aging

"Old age is a strange, blunt foe. And it fights
dirty. It isn't fair."

—Peg – Solos - Season 1

COMPLIANT AGING IS my term. It came about watching how we attack aging. And in a word, most of us don't. We accept what is happening to our bodies as the price of getting older. By compliant, I mean that we compensate for the ravages of aging by changing the way we move and the way we live, instead of the way we age.

Many of you will tell me that I'm wrong. You'd say that even as you age, you stay active. I realize some of you continue to run, swim, walk, or play a sport. Many of you intend to be athletic for as long as possible. Those activities are vital to your long-term fitness but are only a piece of the puzzle. Yes, they are good for you, but they don't attack all the changes that are in motion in your aging body.

I'm going to paint an ugly picture of aging. Our bodies eventually fail all of us, and life always ends in death. We don't have a lot of choice about the ending. Aging happens to different people at different rates. Some people are blessed to arrive at eighty-five or ninety, pretty much intact. Most of us don't fare as well. How we take care of ourselves and how we attack aging can make a significant difference in our quality of life as we get older.

I work out regularly and try to stay as strong and healthy as I can. That said, I know that I could drop dead from a stroke or heart attack tomorrow. I could end up with Parkinson's or cancer or a million other things. What I am talking about won't stop or cure the inevitable. So, why bother, you might ask? Because, with some hard work, the trip through aging can be a little easier to bear, and we can live a higher quality of life while we're here. Even if you get a chronic illness, being strong and fit can help you navigate the changes brought on by that illness. In this chapter, let's look at the impacts of aging if we choose to concede to the tides of time.

You may not think much about aging if you've always been strong and healthy, even without exercise. If that's true, you are one lucky person. Or you've played tennis or golf for years and consider yourself fit. Do you walk three or four miles each week and pat yourself on the back for getting it done? I'm sorry to tell you that aside from good genetics, we are all playing by the same rules, and you will eventually fall to the same ills as the rest of us. Unless you're making a targeted effort to build muscle, you will lose as much as 5 percent of your muscle mass each decade over thirty. As you get older, the rate at which you lose muscle speeds up, and eventually that loss will express itself as weakness.

Not only are you losing muscle, but you're also losing a larger percentage of the muscle fiber that allows you to move quickly. Why do you care? You may need to slam on the brakes at any age, throw a leg out to stop a fall, or catch a grandchild before they run into the road. Have you ever seen a senior who can't walk fast enough to get across the street before the light turns? Although we don't spend much time thinking about it, losing the ability to move quickly can significantly impact our quality of life. Yes, being active may slow down that muscle loss. And activities like tennis may keep you fast and agile. But that doesn't necessarily turn into strength, as you will see from Chuck's story.

When the newly built gym I work at opened up in 2018, Chuck joined because it was convenient and close to home. Chuck is a retired CFO and has been training and taking classes. But let's let him tell his story.

"When my wife retired, our insurance plan switched, and our new insurance included an Anytime Fitness membership. Our local gym was brand-new, so I became a member. At sixty-five, I was running three miles twice a week and played tennis once a week. I considered myself in great shape for my age. How many sixty-five-year-old men can run three miles twice a week? But I was shocked to find that I was losing muscle mass. I could see that loss just by looking at my arms. I was horrified when I realized how little I could bench press in my basement gym. I took an introductory training session when I joined the gym and was stunned to discover just how much strength I'd lost. I also found my balance wasn't as good as I thought it was. The tennis and running made me faster and more agile, and that's always a positive. But it did little to slow muscle loss or to build the muscle I needed to improve my balance and strength."

And muscle mass is the key to aging gracefully and maintaining your independence. Why? Your muscles get you out of a chair and off the bed. They get you into and out of the tub and off the toilet. When you can't do these things for yourself, you can't live independently. You may think you're doing all you can to stay fit as you age, but aging is a complicated process, and there's no one solution.

Let's talk about osteoporosis. You may think the loss of bone density or osteoporosis is something that happens only to women. You would be wrong. Male or female, you can develop osteoporosis as you age. Falls are dangerous, and the fear of falling can be just as dangerous. How can that be? If you become less active because of the fear of taking a serious fall, that inactivity can lead to bone and muscle loss, increasing your chance of being injured if you fall. It becomes a vicious circle.

And thinning bones are no joke. You slow down just a little every time you fall and break a bone. One in two women over fifty will have a fracture related to osteoporosis in their lifetime. And if you're a man, you don't get a free pass. One in five men is at risk for an osteoporosis-related fracture. Don't just skim over those numbers. Next time you go to dinner with the girls, look around. There is a chance that 50 percent of the women at your table will experience a broken bone due to osteoporosis. You want to be in the percentage of people who don't have that experience.

Hip fractures can be devastating, and many who experience a fractured hip never regain the same level of independence they had before the fracture. In the twelve months following an osteoporotic fracture, research indicates a death rate between 20 and 40 percent. There is significant variability between age and sex, but the death rate is frightening, even at its lowest. If you needed no assistance before a hip fracture, there is a better than even chance that you won't be able to get off the toilet or out of a chair without help following that fracture. When you imagine breaking a bone, you think about hard falls or sudden impacts, but a bump on a coffee table can break a leg bone with osteoporosis. Is this the picture you have for your retirement?

Let's move on to our failing balance as we age. We can expect our balance to deteriorate 12 to 14 percent each decade after age fifty. There are many reasons why we have balance issues, including muscle loss, heart disease, illness, medications, and many more. Failing balance is something almost all seniors experience in their lifetimes.

As your balance declines and you become more unsteady, your world becomes smaller. Stairs become your enemy. You might have to move into a single-level home. If it's icy out, you stay home, not out of choice but out of fear of falling. And if you fall once, even without injury, you are more likely to compensate by moving less for fear of another fall. And the cycle continues.

When you consider muscle loss, osteoporosis, and declining balance, it doesn't paint a pretty picture for aging. And when all three raise their ugly heads and become a part of your life, it's frightening. With your balance less than optimal, thinning bones, and a loss of strength and coordination, that little sheet of ice on the sidewalk or front porch stairs can be life-altering.

Let's take a quick look at the mechanics of a fall. Imagine you are age seventy with all three conditions present. You've lost a significant amount of strength and speed from muscle loss, you've been diagnosed with osteoporosis, and you have balance issues. You step out of your front door and slip on a tiny sheet of ice. Your balance is bad, so you can't right yourself and stop the fall. Because you've lost muscle mass, particularly that type of muscle that lets you move quickly, you can't throw a leg out or grasp the door jamb in time to catch yourself. You know what happens when you hit the ground. If you are lucky enough to get away with a few bruises, that's great. However, with osteoporosis, you may end up with a broken hip, arm, or back. That fall can be life-changing.

Case in point, aging isn't a single thing. It is multiple things that are all happening in the last third of our lives. Part of the issue with aging is that we're sure it won't happen to us. We won't be the person who falls and breaks a hip, has terrible balance, or needs help getting out of a chair. It's hard to see yourself as that person at fifty, but as every decade passes, you begin to understand just how devastating compliant aging can be.

Some people believe that if they limit what they do, they can avoid a fall. That may be true, but is that how you want to live your life? I'm sure you've noticed that folks who use this strategy have lives that get smaller and smaller each year. The less you move, the more muscle mass, speed, and bone density you lose. When you add impaired balance to this equation, it becomes a deadly cycle.

Many retirees look forward to spending time with grandkids. Do you want to watch that dream die because you can't keep up with them? Do you want to spend your time worrying about being knocked down by the grandkids or the dog instead of joyfully playing with them? Do you want to sit on the couch and watch them play, or would you rather spend the day with them in a park or on a hike? Compliant aging has a very high price.

As our physical capabilities decline, as we become more isolated from family and friends, and as our dreams fall to the wayside, depression, which is not a normal part of aging, can rear its ugly head. And life just gets harder and harder. With isolation and lack of engagement with the outside world, the old age train picks up speed.

Lack of exercise is only one of the issues we face as we age. Eat a poor diet, load up on sugar, don't exercise, and you may suffer from metabolic syndrome. Metabolic syndrome is a silent condition that includes high blood pressure, high blood sugar, high cholesterol, and excess body fat around your waist. Without lifestyle changes, it can lead to heart disease, stroke, and diabetes, all of which can destroy your retirement quality and lead to an early exit from this earth.

Metabolic syndrome doesn't happen overnight just because you reached a certain age. Based on your lifestyle, it can happen at almost any age. I was most certainly in its grip by my middle fifties. I had high blood pressure and excess fat around my middle. Sometimes, I wonder where I would be if I hadn't discovered resistance training.

I am not trying to oversell the ills of aging. It is a process of decay that goes on for much of our lives. We can't stop aging, but we can manage many of its effects. I know you've earned the right to finally sit down and do as you damn well please, but there is a high price to pay for all that sitting and relaxing.

As you become weaker and slower, combined with failing balance, your life can change significantly. Things you love may fall to the wayside. The up and down of gardening might not be possible. Your best friend has a flight of concrete stairs up to her front door. What if you can't climb those stairs anymore? Did you plan to travel during your retirement years? Do you want to be limited to only those places that don't require much physical effort? Do you know of any great tours that require no walking, climbing, or lifting? I am sure they exist but is that what you want?

As we age, our brain loses track of where our limbs are. Short-term memory goes into hiding. We become impatient, and we can't multitask or do math in our heads like we used to. These changes don't happen overnight, but slowly and surely, our mental faculties begin to decline. My mom had no severe memory issues, but she started getting lost in new places, and one day when she was in her early seventies, she handed me her keys and stopped driving. She had found herself lost in the town she had lived in for twenty-five years and had called me to help her find her way home. Could resistance training have helped maintain her memory? I don't know, but I am sure it wouldn't have hurt and might have allowed her to keep her independence longer.

If you are older than fifty-five or sixty, you know what's happening to your memory. You can lose your keys when they're in your hand. I think we all worry about the more frightening elements of brain health in all the different forms of dementia. Is there anything you wouldn't do to help maintain a healthy brain?

We go from walking to a walker to a wheelchair and assume it's a natural process that happens to everyone. No one teaches us how to maintain our strength and balance. And worse, we don't believe we can do much about how we age, so we do nothing. Our mental and physical health determines our level of independence, and as that fails, so does our ability to live independently.

We retire, take a deep breath, and make plans for the next twenty years. But we take no positive, physical action to make sure our bodies can stay strong and healthy so we can enjoy all those plans we made. That's what I call compliant aging. We just comply. We don't fight back. We don't educate ourselves. We think we're old, and we give up and concede defeat before we've even fought the battle. Why? We give up because we don't truly believe that there is anything we can do to change the trajectory of our lives.

Let's talk about how we compensate as we age. What do I mean by compensating? I'm talking about the changes we make in how we live and move as we begin to feel the effects of muscle loss, bone loss, and failing balance. Have you ever noticed seniors rolling out of a chair? Ever wondered why they do that? Or how they went from healthy and strong to struggling to stand up?

We've already talked about how your ability to get out of a chair, off the toilet, or out of bed determines your level of independence. Those tasks become more difficult as each year passes, and you age and lose muscle mass. What allows you to stand straight up from a chair? It is leg strength, stability, and coordination, and aging impacts all three.

As you're aging, you don't get a memo to let you know that your legs are getting weaker. You may start to change how you stand up by leaning forward and using momentum to get to your feet. It happens so slowly over time that you don't notice. You'll start looking around for chairs with arms that you can push off from, and you can buy toilet rails or special high seats to make standing up easier. You might not sit on the comfy couch that you love because you know you'll sink into those cushions and never get up. Many lawn chairs aren't safe because the arms won't support you when you use them as leverage to stand.

Climbing stairs, getting off the floor—things you used to do with ease—get more challenging over time. These changes happen slowly, but you will notice them the day you can't get off the floor without help. The awkwardness of restaurant booths may force you to stick to tables and chairs. You may even avoid going out with friends for fear of being in a new place where you can't get up without help.

Currently, we have a life expectancy approaching eighty years. That was not true a hundred years ago when life expectancy was closer to fifty-four years. Many of us will have twenty or even thirty years of retirement to spend as we wish. This is what makes understanding how we age so important. Now that you know what aging looks like without intervention, let's move on and find out just how much we can positively impact how we age.

CHAPTER 3

The Magic Bullet

"Take care of your body. It's the only place
you have to live."

—Jim Rohn

HOW CAN EXERCISE, primarily resistance and cardio training, impact aging? First, please don't think of
barbells and heavy lifts when I say resistance training. There are many ways to do effective resistance
training, and we'll cover those in later chapters.
Aerobic exercise or cardio doesn't necessarily mean
the treadmill or elliptical. You have many options for
both forms of training. And when you think of any
kind of exercise, remember that you will start training
wherever you are physically. What you do should be
tailored to your abilities, and if you need to start with
a one-pound weight, then that's where you start. So

please keep an open mind as we move forward. None of this is as complicated as it may sound at first.

Secondly, you want your doctor on board with your program. Your doctor will have insight into your current physical condition, bone density, balance, and coordination. Finding a doctor who was on my team was a challenge, but they are out there. An injury can take you out of the game for a long time, and a referral to a sports medicine doctor can be a lifesaver.

When I go in about a shoulder or a knee, they treat me like an athlete and help me function at the highest level I can. If they send you to physical therapy and send you home with exercises, do them. Starting a fitness program as a senior is one area of life where you're better off asking for permission instead of forgiveness. That said, I will say again, finding a doctor who was on my team was a challenge. You may have to search a bit for the doctor or doctors you need to support your goals.

Let's begin with how you can impact muscle loss. The previous chapter talked about losing muscle mass and fast-twitch muscle fiber. As a reminder, fast-twitch fiber is the fiber that allows you to move quickly. When you use the proper training program, your muscles are damaged at a microscopic level. The process of repair fuses the muscle fibers, building more muscle mass. This training lets you offset some or all of the muscle loss you experience with aging.

Since you lose more of the muscle type that allows

you to move quickly, your workouts should include programming to help you rebuild that muscle fiber. Just think about the senior crossing a busy street. That person may have the strength to get across the street, but can't move fast enough to beat the light. We've all seen that happen. Another example is the ability to throw an arm or leg out quickly to stop a fall. If you have ever fallen and watched the ground come up to meet you, you know what I mean. Building muscle is critical to our ability to stay safe and independent. Building power, which is strength times speed, is just as important.

Rebuilding the muscle fiber that lets you move quickly can be done in several different ways. That "power" work will be a part of your program and can be as simple as a quick knee lift done repetitively, a fast sled push, or a quick step forward or backward. There is a lot of complicated science around how seniors lose muscle with aging. Luckily the science of rebuilding that muscle isn't quite as complex and is within reach of all of us.

Building that muscle can also help to improve balance. A 2014 study in the *Journal of Clinical & Diagnostic Research* compared three groups (Joshua, et al.). One group did traditional balance training. A second did a combination of resistance and balance training. The third group did resistance training, focusing on lower limb strength. The results of the study showed that the resistance training only group showed the most improvement (Joshua, et al., 2014, p. 102). This makes sense since having the strength to stabilize yourself when your balance is an issue is essential. We know that resistance training can improve your stability.

Let's talk a bit more about stability. You are building a bridge. Imagine you make a rope bridge. It may be strong rope, but if you're on this bridge and wind comes up, the bridge will sway. The bridge is not stable. You can't control the wind, but you can control how you build the bridge. Make that bridge steel with a concrete base, and not even a hurricane can move it. You want to be the bridge with those concrete pillars. Regardless of why your balance is an issue, having a strong, solid base will go a long way toward helping you avoid a fall. So resistance training focusing on stability will need to be an essential part of your program. You may see training for balance referred to as balance training or stability training. Both terms are accurate, and stability is what you are after.

What can resistance training do for the last part of the Evil Triad, osteoporosis? You already understand that bone loss or osteoporosis can be an issue for both sexes as we age. And fractures can significantly impact your independence. But resistance training can help here also. In simple terms, our bones bear the weight of our bodies. Resistance training targeting weight-bearing exercises in addition to walking can help you maintain and build bone density. A farmer's carry involves walking or standing with weight in both hands. This weight is borne across your shoulders, down your spine, across your hips, and down your legs. Exactly where you want to build bone. It's also excellent grip training.

Resistance training, walking, any weight-bearing movement is good for your bones. Resistance exercises can vary from simple bodyweight work to farmer's carries and deadlifts. Dancing, walking, sports (playing, not watching them), even work around the house and yard can contribute to your bone health. Anytime you are moving your body weight against gravity, you are strengthening your bones. So for heaven's sake, keep moving!

But there is even more good news! Resistance training also has benefits for your heart. Aerobic activity increases your heart and breathing rate. When you think of aerobic exercise, you may think of running, walking, tennis, biking, or using the treadmill or elliptical in the gym. But many strength training activities also increase your heart and respiration rate. It is anaerobic exercise, which supports bursts of activity.

Full-body exercises like a squat to a press, deadlifts, or pushups will get your heart rate up. If you move quickly between activities, you can get the benefits to your heart much like traditional cardiovascular exercises if you so choose.

A 2019 study showed that resistance training may reduce your risk of heart attack and stroke by 40 to 70 percent (Liu, et al., 2019, p. 499), with only an hour per week of weightlifting. That is huge! The study did not find any additional benefit to your heart for lifting more than an hour per week (Liu, et al., 2019, p. 504). Another study that surveyed 4,000 adults showed that resistance training could be linked to reduced heart disease, and that link was more robust than for those who only walked or cycled (Phillips Smith, et al., 2018). Nothing I read suggested that aerobic activity via walking and cycling did not positively impact one's health. Still, there is support for the addition of resistance training to provide even more protection from cardiovascular disease.

Now I'm going to make a claim you may find hard to believe. Resistance training slows down aging. How? Let's talk about chronological age versus biological age. Chronological age is your age in years. At this writing, I am sixty-five, and that's my chronological age. There are no factors that will let me adjust my chronological age. It is what it is. On my next birthday, I will be one year older regardless of any of my activities.

Biological age takes in multiple factors, including genetics, lifestyle, nutrition, diseases, stress, and smoking. Biological age is about how old we seem, and it can be older or younger than your chronological age. I will use myself as an example. I am an ex-smoker. In my mid-fifties, I was obese, didn't exercise, and I definitely had poor nutrition. My biological age was assuredly higher than my chronological age. If I had stayed on that path, my biological age now would be much greater than sixty-five.

Without dumping a lot of science on you, common sense tells you that managing your bone loss, building muscle mass, training regularly, and eating a healthy diet gives you a younger biological age than someone who chooses compliant aging. I say that as if it is a choice, and in most healthy, active agers, it *is* a choice.

There are tests to calculate your biological age, but for simplicity, the question is, what age do you feel? I don't feel sixty-five. What age do you feel? Are you stronger or weaker than you were a year ago? Are you faster or slower? How do you want to feel this time next year? How is your balance? Have you had a DEXA scan, and do you understand what your current bone density is? Can you do the things around your home that allow you to live independently? Can you get up and down from the floor? Do you have the energy to enjoy every day of your hard-earned retirement? I am simplifying this subject, but I want you to understand that you can impact your biological age with exercise. And you are never too old to start.

Let's look at two imaginary seventy-year-old men who we'll call Joe and Fred. This will be a very high-level comparison. We will not take into account stress, genetics, disease, or nutrition. Neither of our imaginary gentlemen is obese or has any serious illnesses, so they both seem healthy at first glance. Joe hasn't been very active since retirement. He hits the golf course once a week and occasionally takes a walk with his wife. His fitness activities are limited, and he does no serious weight or aerobic training. At seventy, we will assume he's lost 20 percent of his muscle mass. Chances are it could be more than 20 percent, but we'll keep it simple for this example.

Joe is finding that he's a bit slower each year. Walks are getting shorter. Getting out of a chair or off the sofa is difficult, and golf games aren't as much fun as they used to be. What's frustrating him is that he's getting stiff, putting on weight, and running out of energy before the day is over. His chronological age is seventy, and his biological age is at least seventy or higher.

Now let's look at Fred. Fred is also seventy and retired at the same age as Joe. Fred walks two days a week, a mile or more, at a brisk pace. If the weather doesn't allow for a walk, then he's on the treadmill or rower at the gym for at least thirty minutes twice a week. He does weight training twice a week, focusing on leg and back strength, so his muscle mass hasn't declined. Fred plays tennis once a week and has maintained much of the muscle that lets him moves quickly. At the end of each session, he stretches and does a few minutes of mobility. His chronological age is seventy, but Fred looks and feels like a sixty-year-old, so his biological age is sixty. Instead of losing muscle, he's building it, and he is maintaining his range of motion and endurance.

I hope the examples help you to understand just how much impact you can have on your biological age as you get older. This example would be true if the stories were about women. And since women are more inclined to lose bone density, the woman doing aerobic and weight training would most likely have much better bone density than the woman on the couch. Because of the weight training, she would also be more stable and less likely to suffer a life-threatening fall.

You can even improve your brain health with exercise. There is a lot of complicated science out there, but I will simplify this discussion for our purposes. Weight training improves the area of the brain that controls executive function. Executive function allows you to multitask, do math in your head, and, among other things, control your impulses. It sounds like a pretty important area to me.

Resistance training has also been shown to impact memory and provides some protection against dementia. It doesn't seem to prevent dementia or the related diseases like Alzheimer's, but it has been shown to slow the progression. A study published in *NeuroImage: Clinical* studied older people with mild cognitive impairment or MCI (Broadhouse, et al., 2020). The risk of dementia within a year is one in ten for those with MCI. The one hundred participants were separated into four groups. The resistance training groups did ninety minutes of training per week over two or three sessions. Only the two groups, the one who did progressive resistance training (PRT) and the one who did PRT with computerized cognitive training, showed improvement (Broadhouse, et al., 2020, p. 6). I am going to quote this statement as I think it is very compelling.

> "This is the first time any intervention, medical or lifestyle, has been able to slow and even halt degeneration in brain areas particularly vulnerable to Alzheimer's disease over such a long time," said Professor Valenzuela from the Sydney Medical School in the Faculty of Medicine and Health. (Reiner, 2020, para. 15)

So resistance training in itself has benefits that most of us have never considered. The fear of dementia in all its facets is as frightening as any physical issues we might develop. The fact that resistance training is one more tool in our toolbox that might help us maintain a healthy brain makes it worth the effort, regardless of the many other benefits offered.

I think now is the time to introduce Lynn. Lynn is sixty-eight and has been at the gym for over two years. She takes group classes and does personal training one day a week. Lynn both hikes and bikes, so she's an active lady. I asked her how she feels physically after two years of consistent workouts, including strength training. Here is her response.

"When I joined, I hoped to increase joint mobility, maintain if not increase strength (build some muscle if possible at my age), and to continue to work on endurance. If I'm in this for the long haul, I'll need stamina. I also want to maintain balance so I can keep hiking and biking. The classes at my previous gym were more aerobic, and they also had different yoga styles and Pilates. I guess I was kind of expecting those sorts of classes at the new gym. Boy, was I surprised when we used free weights and the suspension training, something I've never done before. And the pushups and burpees, oh my! I didn't think I felt too awful when I first started, but I really notice a difference now after two and a half years with the new gym. Joint mobility is increased. I especially notice improved neck mobility when driving and turning to look over my shoulder for traffic as I'm about to turn. I am definitely stronger, and I've built some muscles. My balance is good; I hike on rocky trails and climb rocks with confidence. I continue to bike and get my 10,000 steps in most days. Also, my latest DEXA scan noted improved bone mass in my spine."

If nothing else I've said has moved you to keep reading, I hope Lynn's story will do just that.

So, let's move on. Before you can start your journey to a new and fitter you, we need to examine some of the myths and ageism you will experience as you begin the *Train to Age* journey.

CHAPTER 4

Myths and Ageism

"Age is no barrier. It's a limitation you put on your mind."

—Jackie Joyner-Kersee

I REMEMBER MY mom telling me that when you get old, people treat you differently. She got my typical eye roll because I knew that probably wasn't the case. Well, that's one of the many things I'll need to apologize for when I get to heaven. People do treat you differently. So, let's begin this discussion by talking about the term "ageism."

Ageism is simply prejudice or discrimination based on a person's age. Have you ever forgotten something and had someone, maybe even family, assume it's your age? I had a doctor tell me I should slow down. He said he was forty-three, and he was already feeling his age. I have no words for comments like that. Telling me to slow down based on how he felt at forty-three is ageism. There is no reason to believe that at sixty-five, I should slow down because he feels old.

Families believe the less you move, the less likely you are to fall and get injured. Our kids love us and want to keep us safe. But the truth is you already know what happens when you become inactive and park yourself on the couch. Do you need to train within your abilities? Of course, you do. Make sure your children also understand the consequences of inactivity and the benefits of movement. Start where you are and slowly move forward. Remember that term "compression of morbidity." Both you and your family want to reduce the amount of time you spend disabled or frail.

I have taught classes where the fittest person in the room was sixty-five-plus, even when many younger folks participated. If you look around and really see people, you'll notice that fitness and age are not related. I've learned not to assume what someone, regardless of age, can or cannot do. I let them tell me if they have limitations.

Have you ever simply glanced at a twenty-year-old and decided what you thought they might be unable to do in a workout? Probably not. I've seen time and again where someone will look at a seventy-year-old and decide their limitations before speaking with them. I've even been guilty of that on occasion myself.

I've met trainers who are afraid of training seniors for fear they will "break."

Getting old is hard enough without society making assumptions based on age. Why is this important? Because when people make assumptions about what a person is capable of based on any single factor—age, sex, race, or gender—discrimination soon follows. Society should not decide what you can or cannot do. You are the only person who determines what your capabilities are.

Have you ever Googled memes about aging? Sure, some are smart, supportive, or funny. But many make old folks look downright stupid, weak, and useless. And a lot of people buy into that picture of aging, including active agers. It's hard to expect more from yourself when it feels like much of society expects nothing.

Active agers are just as varied as any other age group. Some are weak, and some are strong; we vary in temperament and belief. We all have our physical issues since most of us don't get to sixty and beyond without a few bumps and bruises. But our age group is diverse and our capabilities vary widely. It's bad when assumptions are made based on our age, but it's even worse when we believe them. Let's tackle a few myths on aging that we may have begun to believe.

Have you heard that old dogs can't learn new tricks? Have you passed on learning something new just because you believe you are too old? I've seen a lovely seventy-nine-year-old lady learn to deadlift and slam battle ropes. We call her Battle Rope Betty, and she's one big smile when she's at the gym. Although initially there was some hesitation when I added deadlifting to some of my senior group classes, I have never had a student who couldn't learn and didn't benefit from increased self-confidence and strength regardless of the weight on the bar. I don't recall any of my students being unable to learn a new skill or exercise. A new piece of equipment might cause a little trepidation until they get the form down, and then off they go. Do I make modifications based on their age and physical ability? Sure I do. That has nothing to do with their ability to learn new things. I definitely wouldn't tell Betty that old dogs can't learn new tricks. She might just pop you with her battle rope!

Another myth that I frequently hear is that you shouldn't exercise or you might get injured. I understand and agree that you don't want to get injured as an active ager. The older you are, the longer it takes for injuries to heal. There is also the fear that an injury will be severe enough to impact your ability to stay independent, and no one wants to ask for help, regardless of age. But we already know the outcome if you don't exercise, and it's not pretty. The trick is to start training where you are and to carefully move forward from there.

The truth is, if you don't build strength, power, endurance, mobility, and stability, you WILL eventually get injured. We don't spontaneously get stronger by wishing it. Biologically though, we do get weaker as we age. So, if you want to avoid injury, you have to fight back, and you do that by maintaining and building the physical abilities that are beginning to fail. That Evil Triad is always there waiting, just around the corner. Exercise, including targeted training, is one way to fight back. Good genetics and health may get you farther down the road, but targeted training can help you hold the line regardless of when you start.

You will ease into your Train to Age program, and you'll do it with an eye on keeping safe. You can train at whatever level is appropriate for you. If you haven't worked out in forty years and have led a sedentary lifestyle, please don't jump back in like you're a twenty-year-old. You're not. I will say this again and again. Start where you are and move forward from there. Jump in and train like a kid, and your body will quickly remind you that you are no longer that twenty-year-old. Starting your program with too much intensity is a great way to convince yourself you are old and you can't do this. Give yourself a chance and start slow. I know you know that slow and steady wins the race.

Let's move on to myth number three. I've had people tell me that you should never pick up a weight heavier than ten pounds when you're older. I've had to work hard to convince some of my female clients that you can safely move up in weight. The fear of injury sometimes stops them in their tracks. If there are overriding medical issues, of course, this might be true. There are conditions and illnesses where taking great care with weight is necessary. But without some specific reason, it makes no sense to put an arbitrary number on what an active ager should lift. You start light and work your way up as you get stronger. This isn't a race, so you increase weight at your own pace.

But in the larger sense, we active agers carry in groceries, climb stairs, carry dog food, cat food, and sometimes grandkids. I've carried mulch and topsoil, and I'm glad for the strength I have. Picking your body up out of a chair takes strength, and your legs are lifting more than ten pounds when you stand. There are many instances where we need to pick up something that weighs more than ten pounds in real life. Avoiding resistance training doesn't make sense if you want to stay independent and injury-free.

If you find working with weights a bit frightening, then think more about what you physically want to be able to do. Carrying a grandchild or a suitcase requires enough strength to move their weight. Getting out of a chair or up the stairs requires the strength to move your bodyweight through those motions. Walking through a big box store or taking a tour of the city requires you have the endurance to cover a long distance without running out of energy. So instead of worrying about how much weight you should be using, focus on your goals and slowly work up in weight and distance until you can do the things you want to do.

Let's take a look at another myth. To be old is to be frail. Really? Who wrote that rule? So at sixty, you should give up and give in to the inevitable, or is the magic age seventy or eighty? Yes, you might be frail at the end of life, especially from a long-term illness or extreme old age, but no rule says you will be frail at a specific time in your life. And no one wants to spend the last twenty or thirty years of their life as an invalid. Remember the term, compression of morbidity? The whole goal of training is to shorten the time you are frail. You want that time as short and close to the end of your life as you can get it.

You can impact your rate of aging, and you can fight back against the Evil Triad. You can stay strong and independent if you keep moving, keep training, and make that investment in your body that will carry you through the last third of your life. Be assured, before you finish this book, you'll have clear instructions on what you can do to stay strong, and you'll have many options and ways to get that accomplished. So hang in here a bit longer, and we'll soon get the chapter with the answers.

Here's an almost deadly myth. Don't move fast; you'll get hurt. Have you ever seen a person who can't get across the street before the light changes? That looks pretty dangerous to me. Have you ever seen someone fall slowly? No? You haven't because accidents happen quickly and without warning. You have to move fast enough to respond to the danger, whether it's a changing light or a spot of ice on the ground.

We need to do things quickly regardless of age, like hit the brakes, grab the toddler at the top of the stairs, or move out of the way of a moving vehicle. As you age, you lose an excessive amount of muscle fiber that lets you move quickly; a training program that builds back some of that fiber is the answer.

Power training at sixty-five or seventy does not resemble power training for a twenty-year-old. I'm not suggesting box jumps and sprints. Power training is targeted to the skills that will keep you safe, like quickly stepping forward, back, or to the side so that when, in real life, you need to move quickly, you can do so. There are simple drills and exercises you can do to get faster. These exercises should be targeted toward your goals and tailored to your fitness level. Regardless of where you are right now, you can do the work to slow the loss of the muscle fiber that makes you fast without putting your safety at risk.

Some of that power work is about reconnecting your brain to a specific movement. One of the drills I do is the "clock drill." You pretend that you are standing in the middle of a clock face. Midnight is directly behind you, and six o'clock is in front of you. The other hours are in their respective positions on the clock face. I call out a specific time, and the challenge is to quickly shift your weight and tap that time with one foot then return to the starting position.

With most clients, in the beginning, the challenge is getting that brain-body connection rebuilt so you can step without having to take seconds to think about it. The second challenge is then to quickly and safely step and return. Why do this? In real life, when you lose your balance or are trying to avoid an obstacle on the ground, you want both the brain-body connection and the speed to prevent a fall or injury.

To build speed and power (strength times velocity), you don't have to train high-impact moves. You can simply do drills like quick stand-ups or squats. A speed drill can be something as simple as a fast knee lift or step up. The point is, you will train speed in a manner and style that works for you and is safe. The whole point of speed drills is to make sure you can move quickly when the need arises.

Here's the myth that irritates me the most, and there are several versions of it. One version asks, "Why can't you just enjoy what's left of your life?" Another version says, "You're retired; you don't have to do anything you don't want to." I will concede that, like all myths, there is a grain of truth to this one. And for this myth, the truth is you don't *have* to do anything you don't want to. And this is a time to enjoy life. The other truth is if you don't take care of your body, you won't get to enjoy your retirement for as long as you might like. The point of training is to make sure you get to enjoy these retirement years to the fullest. Why wouldn't you want to do that?

How about the myth that says if you've never learned to exercise, it's too late now. Really? I started resistance training in my late fifties. My home had always been the treadmill on the rare occasions when I spent time at the gym. I was never comfortable in the gym, especially with all those people who looked fit and strong. I was terrified and knew I looked like an idiot. I was always lost and felt uncomfortable and clumsy. I'm still awkward, but now I'm old enough not to care. No one's opinion will keep me out of the gym, even though I still feel clumsy some days. I know there is too much at risk for me to let someone else's opinion stop me from training.

It is a challenge to start exercising, whether you've never done it or it's just been a long time. But I promise you, start slowly and take your time. Be good to your body, and don't worry about what anyone thinks. The only thing that matters is you do the work and live long and prosper. Sorry, I couldn't help myself.

What about the fear of injury? I'm talking now about *your* fear of injury. First of all, talk to your doctor and find out what activities are safe for you. As I've said before, work with a professional who can help you get to your goals without injury. A good training program isn't going to throw you to the sharks. It should start you with activities you can manage safely. Work with someone you trust. I am going to say that again...work with someone you trust!

In the long run, family and even our doctors are

just trying to protect us. That's why finding a program or trainer who has experience training our age group is so important. You need to find someone to start your training where you are physically and move you forward one step at a time. Training for the rest of your life isn't a sprint; it's a never-ending marathon. And if you are comfortable in the gym or a class, then go for it. Every step forward on your fitness journey will get easier.

And training can be uplifting, joyful, surprising, and powerful. Why would you want to miss out on all the fun? The next chapter is where we begin to get into the thick of things. In chapter five, you will learn to *Train to Age*, so turn the page and see what's next!

CHAPTER 5

Training for Results

"The only impossible journey is the one you never begin."

—Tony Robbins

YOU ARE GOING to train for results. What does that mean? You are training to slow or reverse what's happening to your body as you age and to maintain your quality of life. You are not aging along one dimension, so you can't train only one dimension. You're not just losing muscle strength. Your brain is aging, your balance is failing, your bones are thinning, and you're getting a little bit slower and stiffer every year. Wow, that sounds awful every time I read it. To combat those losses, you need to put together a training program to help build strength, speed, and stability. And your programming should help you maintain your bone density and flexibility.

Training to age isn't a one-size-fits-all path. You create your programming based on your health, experience with exercise, and what classes and gyms you can find locally or virtually. You need to explore and find things you enjoy. I can't emphasize that enough. "Enjoy" may not be the right word, but you have to do activities that you are willing to stick with over time. If you give something a try and three months later you still hate every minute of it, it's time for a change.

I don't always enjoy what I am doing, but I always do things that give me the benefits I seek. I tolerate battle ropes, medicine ball slams, squat jumps, and sled pushes because they keep my heart strong and my endurance up for the activities I enjoy, like kettlebells, heavy lifts and the occasional mud run.

You can put your program together in a way that works for you. I started with barbells and have moved on to kettlebells. I wouldn't say I like kickboxing or step class, but I like them much better than spending time on the treadmill, and I've learned to like the elliptical. I get bored quickly, so I use lots of different tools to get all my programming in.

You may be like me and need lots of tools to stay engaged with your fitness routine. Or, you may just want someone to give you programming, and you are fine doing that programming for months at a time. Do what works for you.

During covid quarantine, I trained kettlebells with Carol, a friend and a client. Since the gym was closed and it was spring weather, training outside was possible. With kettlebells, we could get some exercise in despite the quarantine, and it didn't take a lot of equipment. That's one of my favorite things about kettlebell training. If you have a couple of kettlebells, you can get a workout done. The great thing about kettlebells is that you can train strength, speed, stability, and endurance. I find them to be one of the most versatile tools in the gym or at home.

One of my clients, Lynn, very quickly took to kettlebell training. But I'll let her tell you about it. "The kettlebell intrigued me. I especially like the flow sequences using a kettlebell, moving through a series of movements. With the kettlebell, I can get a whole-body workout and elevate my heart rate in a relatively short time. Also, the idea of learning something new helps challenge me mentally."

There are thousands of different ways for you to accomplish all your training. If it's been a while since you've walked into a gym or taken a group class, you'll find that variety is alive and well in the fitness world. Of course, the only way to explore that variety is to give new things a try. Regardless of your physical starting point, there is something out there for everyone. We'll talk more about options later in the book. For right now, keep reading and learning, and don't give up.

If you are one of those folks who walk three days a week, then kudos for staying active, but you are missing essential pieces of your training if that's your entire program. If you go to the gym and make one run through the machines and consider yourself done, you still have more work to do. You are working out to add to or to maintain your quality of life. As you go on your journey, don't forget that's the goal. If you hike, golf, play tennis, or practice yoga or tai chi, good for you. But all those activities are only part of the story.

Strength is the starting place for everything. Without it, nothing else really matters. Let's talk about progressive resistance training (PRT). This is a long phrase for a simple concept. To gain strength and muscle mass, your muscles must move against some type of resistance, and as you get stronger, you need to increase the resistance. You don't have to lift heavy to get results. You simply add a little more weight to a movement when the weight you are using isn't yielding strength. When the weight is boringly simple to work with, it's time to move up in weight a bit.

For example, to train your bicep, you might do bicep curls with five-pound weights. With consistent training, that five-pound weight will become too comfortable. You won't be sore, you won't be tired, and more importantly, you won't get results when it becomes too easy. When that happens, you increase your weight, which allows you to continue to stimulate muscle growth and build strength. You increase the weight slowly but steadily over time as you get stronger.

Here's another example. Let's suppose you are seventy years old and are struggling to get out of a chair. You may start training by simply standing up ten times. Your trainer may use a higher seat to make it easier to get started. We have a jump box at my gym that works well for stand-ups because it's a few inches taller than a traditional chair, making it easy to stand up. When standing up becomes more comfortable, you may use a lower seat or grab a weight. As you practice standing with weight, standing up without weight becomes more manageable. If you move well, you might do bodyweight squats. Those are squats using only your body as resistance. As you get stronger, you add weight to make it more difficult. All of these different steps build leg strength. Leg strength gets you to your goal of standing up with ease.

Don't be the person who runs through all the machines in the gym and never increases the weight. Over time, you must increase the weight you are using if you want your body to respond. Failure to increase weight is one of the most common mistakes I see. You don't have to increase it by a lot, but you have to incrementally increase the weight you are using to yield results.

If you have bad knees, which many of us do, you can still train leg strength without causing significant knee pain, so don't stop reading yet. Suspension training uses straps with handles connected to a bar or held by a door, allowing many of my clients with knee pain to do squats pain-free because of the support. Marching in a seated position with or without leg weights can help build leg strength, usually without knee pain. There are many ways to train leg strength, even with bad knees. Why do I keep talking about leg strength? You have to be able to walk, stand, and get out of bed or up from a chair if you want to maintain your independence. It is your number one priority. The good news is that there are many ways to build that strength.

You progress at your own pace, but you must continue to move forward. How do you know you're not getting results? If the muscle you're working isn't feeling tired after three sets, you may need to increase your weight. If you are never sore in any way, you might need to increase your weight. If you can easily do more than sixteen to twenty repetitions without breaking a sweat, you might need to increase your weight. You want to be able to do ten to sixteen repetitions of the movement and feel like you've worked, but you've not strained or become injured. And slow and steady is the rule when you're working with weight.

Remember I said to start where you are? In the beginning, you might only be able to do five or six repetitions. That's fine; next week, do one more rep. You work at your own pace. I spend time in group classes making sure my clients are not comparing themselves to others in the class. Our bodies have all been on separate journeys regardless of age, and making comparisons is fruitless and sometimes leaves us feeling defeated. Your *Train to Age* journey belongs only to you. Make it your own and forget about comparing yourself to the other guy. In the long run, they don't matter. Someone who is seventy and fit but doing nothing to maintain strength, balance, and muscle mass moves backward. Make sure you are moving forward.

I want to introduce you to one more concept. That concept is specificity. It means you train for what you are trying to get better at. If you want to get out of a chair more easily, you train by getting out of a chair or doing squats or some movement to help you get out of a chair and build leg strength. If you have difficulty climbing a flight of stairs, you might do step-ups. That would be stepping up and down from a step. The height on many step boxes is adjustable, so you can start with a lower step and raise it as you get stronger. You train for the problem you are trying to solve, in addition to general fitness. Make sure your training is tailored to you and is effective. That will allow you to get back to the important things in your life.

If you train a specific skill like rising from a chair, be sure and consider how you will measure success. After a few months of training, is it easier for you to get out of a chair? Are you able to get up and down off the toilet better than you could before you started to train? If one of your goals at the gym is simply to walk farther after training than you can when you start, then measure it. How far can you comfortably walk when you begin training compared to how far you can walk after three to six months of training? If you do not see improvement, then it's time to change up your program.

Next, let's talk about power. Power is force times velocity. Think about swinging a baseball bat. The faster the bat moves when it connects with the ball, the farther that ball will go. Remember when you were young, and you could just pop up out of a chair? Now getting up may be a slower process. You may even roll forward to throw some momentum into standing. This loss of speed expresses itself in many different ways as we age. Maybe you've seen something fall off a counter and hit the floor because you just weren't fast enough to catch it.

Have you ever seen the person who can get up from a chair but does it so slowly you wonder if it's ever going to happen? Have you noticed you're, very literally, slowing down? Not long ago, I decided to take a step class on the video system at our gym. My first thought was *Well, this will be fun!* As much as I know about aging, I was surprised to find myself just a hair behind the teacher all the time, and I couldn't catch up! It was very irritating. I have since done the class enough to keep up, but I have a much better understanding of what happens as we lose that fast-twitch muscle fiber. Moving fast enough to do a step class is work. It was much easier ten years ago.

When you think about power training, I don't want you to think about violent movements. We're not talking box jumps here. Just as there are many ways to do strength training, there are many different ways to do power training.

I want to be fast when I need to, so I do power training. That may be doing squats, where I go down slowly and come back up very quickly. I use an agility ladder in some of my classes. You can do fast knee lifts, quick stands, line drills, and if you are so inclined, you can do vertical and lateral jumps, line hops, and fast feet. Just remember that the list is endless and should be tailored to your fitness level. You can rebuild some of the speed that you've lost. Of course, if you play any kind of racquet sport, you probably have maintained your ability to move quickly. Your goal may be to increase your muscle mass. As with everything else, you start where you are and move forward.

You'll hear me repeatedly say that no single activity is enough to overcome the physical losses you are experiencing. We lose abilities across multiple dimensions. We need to train across multiple dimensions if we want to stay as fit as possible, so our next point of discussion is endurance training. Why is endurance training necessary? You may have the strength to walk but can't walk through a big box store without resting. Maybe you can't climb stairs or take a vacation that includes walking long distances or climbing hills. Sometimes, it's as simple as performing activities around your home without being exhausted after each task.

Endurance training as an active ager is about your personal goals and no one else's. I worked with one client in her eighties who simply wanted to walk around the block and visit her neighbors like she did when she was younger. As she aged, the distance she could go without having to stop and rest got shorter and shorter. Instead of visiting with her neighbors, she ended up waving at them across her driveway. How did we train? We walked as far as she comfortably could at each session. We always tried to go a little farther each time. Regardless of your goal, it's an important goal because it's important to you. Don't let anyone tell you otherwise.

Every single person is different and has to figure out what their goals are. Endurance is one area where a trainer might help. You don't have to use a trainer, but they can evaluate your fitness level and develop an incremental training plan to get you where you want to be. The general rule is to increase the activity a little at each workout. One of my clients starts each training session by increasing the distance she walks on the treadmill each time she trains. It's a slow process, but it's a win for both of us when she tells me she can walk her dog a little farther each week.

We have a kettlebell club at my gym, and we train

lots of different things, but often we work on high-volume swings, cleans, and snatches. I am so proud of my clients when they complete a task like 200 swings that they thought they weren't capable of. You are capable of so much more than you think you are. You can do endurance training with a specific goal in mind or work toward general fitness goals. Can anyone guarantee that you'll get to your goals? No. But I can guarantee that you won't if you don't try. Give yourself a chance.

Let's move the discussion to balance. Some people have outstanding balance into their seventies or eighties; most of us are not that lucky. As we've discussed before, there are multiple reasons why our balance degrades. Sometimes it happens so slowly you don't realize it's happening until you trip or take a fall. For this discussion, I would like to focus on building stability. Why? I can't correct the medical reasons for poor balance. I *can* train strength and speed to help minimize the impact of failing balance.

One definition of stability is the ability to remain balanced and not fall. That is precisely what we're trying to do. A primary goal of your training will be to build a good, stable base. Combining stability with speed allows you to catch yourself before you fall, and working on core strength lets you return your body to an upright position if you lose your balance.

How do you train stability? Resistance training naturally builds stability. As you strengthen your glutes, core, and legs, you become more stable. This training in itself will do much to keep you in an upright position. Adding single-leg stands that include a strong core, glutes, and a solid supporting leg will help build stability. Your goal may simply be to hold your foot up for thirty seconds, one minute, or longer. If your balance is an issue, make sure you have something close at hand to grasp when you are training. When it comes to balance, training safely is number one.

You can also include training to help with your lower body coordination. You can step on, around, or over targets. You can practice control with an agility ladder. There is no end to the ways you can rebuild your coordination to be less impacted by poor balance. I am surprised by how much all my clients enjoy the agility ladder even when they don't move quickly.

I have one client who started taking group classes a few months ago. She always stayed close to a tall box that she could hold on to when she worked out. Slowly but surely, as she got stronger and as we did stability drills, she moved farther and farther away from that box, and today, she doesn't need it at all. That improvement was all she needed to make group classes a priority on her schedule. Simple skills like the ability to move well without feeling unbalanced are sometimes lost as we age. But with work, they don't have to be lost forever.

Your goals are your own, but in my opinion, stability and resistance training combined will do much to help protect you from a fall. Feeling more stable will help quell the fear of falling, which is a definite improvement in your quality of life. It's hard to enjoy yourself when you feel like you're going to take a tumble with your every step. And so many activities go to the wayside as a consequence of that fear. Nothing is more life-affirming than self-confidence in movement. Exactly how to train is coming up, so don't despair. Right now, we're just looking at the dimensions of training at a high level.

Our last dimension of training is mobility. Mobility is simply the ability to move freely and easily. I often see it negated as crucial for active agers, but if you haven't lost range of motion, why give it up without a fight? We get stiffer as we get older, and if you are of an age, you're aware of that. What you might not know is that if you don't work your joints through their full range of motion, you risk losing some of that range. I work with healthy, active agers who struggle to get their arms up over their heads. When the mobility is lost, so is the strength for that movement.

Without activity, ankles get stiff (your base for balance and walking), and knees lose range of motion, as do hips and shoulders. Adding mobility to your training is an easy way to keep your joints fluid. If you have arthritis or stiff joints, mobility training will help you keep the range of motion you have and may even provide improvements.

Now is the perfect time to introduce you to Jan and John. They are both seventy-five years old and have been working out at the gym since it opened. They use their time at the gym to improve all the dimensions of training. For them, their primary focus is on strength and mobility. Jan and John both discovered that they work harder in a group class than they do independently, so both have signed up for our group classes two days a week. Jan's focus is strength, and she is constantly working on mobility in her knees and shoulders. John discovered that he needed more leg strength and more flexibility in both his shoulders and hips. Also, his balance was failing, so those areas are his main focus. Jan finds time to ride the bike at the gym in addition to her group training.

They are both very different people and have different needs for training, but both benefit from training all five dimensions. Each individual will have specific areas where they may need to be more focused, but since all five dimensions are failing, they all need to be a part of your program.

Be creative with your training. Training to Age is a lifelong project that will impact every day of the last third of your life. There will be days you just don't feel like it. Do it anyway. There will be times when you feel like gains are coming too slowly. Remember, if you are not moving forward, you're moving backward. Sometimes you will just be holding your own. That's okay.

The *Train to Age* program isn't magic. I'm not going to tell you that you can get fit in ten minutes a day. I am going to tell you it's completely doable. Let's face it; you're retired. One of the things you have is time. If you can find three hours a week, you will see results. Those three hours can be put together in many different ways. You could work out thirty minutes a day for six days. You can split your week up in any way that works for you as long as you cover all the dimensions. I want you to build a plan that works for you. When it stops working, I want you to have the flexibility to change it up and keep it working for you till the end of the line.

Now that you know the different dimensions you need to train, let's look at how you can build your programming.

CHAPTER 6

Training, Tools, and More

"What seems impossible today will one day become your warm-up."

—Unknown

YOU HAVE INFORMATION about what you need to do. I bet that about now, you're shaking your head and wondering how you're supposed to do it. You might be thinking that it's all too complicated. You might even be wondering if it's going to be worth it. Please hang in there. It will be worth it, and building a program isn't as hard as it sounds right now. Options will be as varied as using a gym, hiring a trainer, joining a park program, working out with friends, and training virtually. We're going to talk about all the different choices you have, so let's get started.

I suggest training one hour, three days a week, or

any combination that gives you three hours in total. You will do two or possibly even three strength training sessions. You will be building stability each time you do legs or core. You'll want to find a trainer or class, either in person or virtual, that allows you to build strength and muscle mass slowly. Here is where you also get the benefits for your heart and brain.

You'll want one endurance session. It could be anything that lets you go farther or push a little harder each time. You could walk, bike, use a treadmill or elliptical. To train endurance, you can work on increasing time, distance, or intensity. You might take an aerobics class. You'll find aerobics classes come in many styles and levels. Many pools have adult lap swims where you can work on endurance and do so in a joint-friendly environment.

I include mobility at the end of all my group classes, so you may discover it as part of a class or when working with a trainer, or you might add a yoga class to your schedule. Chair yoga is an option if you're not quite ready for a regular yoga class.

Remember what I said about power training. For the active ager, this is not box jumps or quick, jerky movements. Weight machines aren't great for power training for older adults either.

Trainers who work specifically with active agers and classes designed for active agers are where you will most likely find power training. Power training is something you may have to look for, or you might find it automatically built into your strength training classes.

Your ticket to success is using the program and tools that keep you active and engaged. My first suggestion is to join a gym. If going to the gym is not your thing, don't stop reading. There are many other ways to train. Why the gym? Most gyms have options for different strength equipment you can use. There might be dumbbells, barbells, medicine balls, suspension training, balance balls, and so on. It's a long list, and that's good news. Having cardio and strength training equipment in one place is an extra benefit.

Doing the same thing day in and day out gets boring. You're trying to build a daily habit, and being bored won't help you get that accomplished. Learning how to use various equipment in the gym will make working out fun and challenging. You don't want to be the person who does a couple of rounds on the machines and goes home because you don't know what else to do. That's a recipe for deciding this getting fit business isn't working.

So, I have two recommendations. The first is to find that gym, and the second is to hire a trainer. Yes, trainers are expensive. But if you can find a good trainer who can get you started on your journey, teach you how to do resistance training safely, get you motivated, and help you build a lifelong habit, that person is worth the price. Talk to your trainer about the five dimensions of training and ask if he or she can incorporate them into your plan. Remember, you're creating a lifestyle, not a hobby. Trainers are not required, but a good trainer will get you started down the right path.

If you're like many active agers, you might have knee or hip replacements or osteoporosis. You could have heart issues, COPD, diabetes, or a million other different problems. *Train to Age* is a long-term investment in your life, and a trainer can help you train safely and effectively. None of those issues mean you can't train. You just have to train safely with the conditions you have. If you have a chronic illness, poor balance, or osteoporosis, check with your doctor before starting a program.

In some cases, you can hire a trainer to come to your home. They may bring equipment, or you may have equipment. That may be a solution for you. It doesn't provide the social connection gyms or classes do, but it's an option.

A good trainer will start by evaluating your fitness level and mobility. They should be willing to discuss your goals and expectations. If you have specific physical issues, ask how they would approach strength training considering your health. If you worry about training because your balance is bad, ask how they handle balance issues. Let them know you also want to train stability, power, mobility, and endurance. Ask how they might incorporate those dimensions into your training.

Someone who has worked with active agers will have answers to your questions and probably good ideas about how you can train for all the dimensions and learn different equipment to keep you engaged. There are many ways to do programming. I have clients I train one day a week but provide programming for two more workouts they can do independently. Another option is to mix training with classes. You can put your programming together in a million different ways. But what if hiring a trainer isn't an option?

Group classes are great as an adjunct to training or instead of a trainer. There are many different types of group classes. You'll find them at gyms, private studios, senior centers, and park districts. There are group classes for everything. You'll find dance, boxing, and cycling. You'll encounter resistance training with lots of different equipment, and you'll find yoga and mobility classes. You may be ready for a regular group class. When I say regular, I mean a class not explicitly designed for active agers. Ages in my "regular" group classes range from twenty year-olds to eighty year-olds.

The easy part is finding classes, and the hard part is finding one that's a fit for you. When I started working out, I was in no shape to take high-powered cardio or resistance classes. I will say this many times; start where you are and then move forward into more challenging training and classes. Many group classes will offer individual modifications for their clients;

you just have to ask. I rarely teach a class where I am not providing modifications for more than one person in attendance. Again, you just have to ask.

Some major hospitals have classes for active agers, as do many senior centers. There is no limit on choices. Group classes, in general, are less expensive than trainers, but there is less room for individuality. If you are looking at group classes, you need to find the ones that work for you and your current fitness level.

In some hospital-supported gyms and senior center settings, you may find programming specifically to improve balance and mobility. Take time to find the classes that give you the benefits you need. In these situations, you may also find chair classes as well as many beginner through advanced classes. Many metropolitan areas have park districts that offer classes in addition to their sports and recreation programs. Park district classes are generally affordable, but park districts aren't everywhere. Many facilities will let you try a free class to see if it's a fit, or they will have trainers on staff to help you determine which environments will work best for you.

But what if you can't find something that works for you? The issue could be financial, or there may not be what you are looking for near you. Working out at home is an option, and you have lots of choices there too. There are many fitness apps for your tablet, phone, and computer. Most require some kind of subscription, but many give you lots of options for different class types. Your smartwatch subscription may offer workouts too.

Companies like Daily Burn, Beachbody, and Les Mills have hundreds of classes from beginner to advanced. You can take them on your computer, tablet, or cast to your TV. The many classes they offer include strength, yoga, and cardio. Some companies, like Les Mills, have specific equipment for their classes that can be purchased. They are not strictly offering active ager workouts, but you will find a great deal of variety in many of these online companies. The companies above are for example purposes. Search online, and you'll be amazed at what you will find.

SilverSneakers classes may be accessible to you through your health insurance. You can go to their website and check your eligibility. Even if it's not available, you can sign up as a fan and use their video library, which at this writing offers 200 workout videos. If SilverSneakers is available to you, in addition to the videos, they have tons of other classes on their website. These classes are designed for active agers and have many options from beginner to advanced and range from yoga to Zumba to strength and cardio workouts. They are a great option if you're training from home.

Curtis Adams, vitalityfl.com, has workouts you can access from his website and his YouTube channel. His workouts specifically target active agers. YogaAnytime is a subscription service that offers yoga and meditation. HASfit (Heart and Soul Fitness) has many free workouts on YouTube for all different fitness levels, including chair workouts. They also have an app you can download to your phone or tablet. You can subscribe to the programs that best meet your fitness goals. It may take some time to find what works for you.

There are too many options for me to cover them all in this book. You'll have to search for what's near you, both physical and virtual. Many places offer free classes or free trial memberships so that you can check out all they offer. There are unlimited options out there; you just have to find the ones that help you meet your goals and that you enjoy. You do not have to spend your time hating what you are doing. The choices are endless.

Having a workout partner can help you up your game. You may not feel like working out on a specific day, but you'll go anyway if you have a friend expecting to work out with you. Group classes allow you to build relationships, and that, in turn, makes your workouts more fun.

Let's review your choices. If you are already familiar with working out in a gym and using various equipment, joining a gym may be a perfect choice. If you can afford a trainer either for the long term or just to help you build out your programming, that's where I would start. One choice is to do both personal and group training. Remember you have three hours per week to cover, and individual training sessions may come in as small an increment as thirty minutes.

What if you can't afford a gym membership or a trainer? You may be in an area where you can find classes through your local senior center or park district. If that's not an option, there is always virtual training online. Look for the activities that suit your fitness level, and remember to stay safe. You want to slowly move forward, building out the dimensions of Train to Age and becoming a better and stronger you each day.

So how do you cover all your bases? That takes planning, and planning is what the next chapter is all about.

CHAPTER 7

Taking on the Challenge

"Start where you are. Use what
you have. Do what you can."

—Arthur Ashe

I HOPE BY now you are all in. You are ready to start moving toward a stronger and more fit you. But I realize I have just buried you in tons of information. You know why you need a training program and understand the benefits. So, what's next? Training to Age is your new job, so let's look at preparing to take on the challenge.

Everything successful requires planning. You know the goal is three hours or 180 minutes of training per week. You could train for thirty minutes six days a week. Four forty-five-minute sessions will work, as will three one-hour sessions. You need at least two sessions of resistance training with a day between them. On your resistance training days, you are building strength, speed, and stability. Your cardio days might include walking, running, biking, dancing, or step. The list is truly endless.

If three hours a week seems like too much to start, then decide what works for you. You can work up to the three hours, so start where you are. I have clients who need the shorter thirty-minute workouts and some who thrive on much longer experiences. Every person is unique.

If you haven't exercised in a long time, then go for the thirty-minute sessions to start. A regular exercise schedule is something you will want to build out slowly. You are building a lifestyle, and that doesn't happen overnight. If you have trouble finding classes or training that is thirty minutes in length and have to do longer sessions, then make sure you have a day of rest between each strength session. You can truly put this together in a way that works for you and your current fitness level.

Your first goal is to plan when you will work out. Don't leave it till the end of the day if you can avoid it. After a long day, it's hard to find the energy to hit the gym, take a class, or exercise with a trainer. When you plan your time, remember you will need time to warm-up and cool down in addition to working out. Decide what days and times you're going to set aside for your program. If you find three hours a week too much to start with, do less. This program is always about doing what works for you. As you get stronger, add another day. But don't lose sight of your goals here. You are investing in your future.

Be willing to do a lot of exploration. It may take time for you to find what works for you. If you take an hour class and it's too much, then find a shorter one. If what you're doing isn't challenging, then look around for something that's a better fit.

Next, think about what you're going to do each day. Your resistance days should have a day of non-resistance between them. Pick your two endurance/cardio days. Whatever makes you move your body and gets your heart rate up will qualify. You have a lot of flexibility with your mobility. You'll find yoga and mobility exercises for active agers online, at your gym, or in classes in your community. Tai chi improves both balance and mobility, and it's very relaxing. I usually start and end my workouts with mobility. Mobility may be a part of your workouts, separate workouts, or both.

I have been asked if it's okay to work out in ten-minute segments instead of a full half hour. If you have to, then it will have to do. But, if you can't find one thirty-minute time period to work out, I don't think there is much of a chance you'll find three separate ten-minute segments to work out either. That said, something is always better than nothing. You could work out three days a week for an hour if that

works for you. You will be putting your workouts together a little differently to get all the dimensions
covered in fewer sessions. Take your time building
your schedule, and make sure it is truly something
you can stick with. It's your schedule, and my only
suggestion would be to avoid putting your strength
days back-to-back.

Now that you have your time blocked out and you
know what you are looking for, you can start your research. Check out your local gyms, classes, and virtual classes. Start where you are. Start slow. You can
move forward from there.

Frustration is easy if you start at a level that's too
hard. I promise, if you keep to your schedule, you will
see improvement. But if you jump into a class that either hurts you or leaves you so sore, you can't move,
that's not a win. Be good to yourself and give yourself
a chance to be successful.

Once you've made the big decisions—what,
when, and where—now you start digging into the de-
tails. Make gyms work for your business. Most will
offer a free trial, walk you through their offerings, and
schedule you to meet with staff.

I will tell you now; most are trying to sell personal
or group training. They know your chance of being
successful without some guidance isn't good. If you
have no experience with resistance training, gym
equipment, or weights, a trainer may be a great way
to start. That said, you have this book, and you have

choices. Make good ones. If you choose to use a personal trainer, here are some things to think about:

1. Does the trainer have experience working with active agers?

2. If you have issues specific to you—replacement parts, diabetes, balance issues, osteoporosis, or any other physical issues—ask if the trainer has any specific thoughts about how they would train you.

3. The trainer will test your strength during the initial free evaluation. They should not push you to a point you feel unsafe. They should also not push you hard just to prove how badly you need them. That said, when you select a trainer, you do want them to challenge you and help you build strength, power, mobility, endurance, and balance.

4. Is the gym clean, and is the floor clear of hazards?

5. Does the trainer have any certifications for training active agers or people with specific training needs?

6. Follow your gut. If you choose to work with a trainer, you need to trust them. They will be balancing keeping you safe and challenging you.

If you decide to try out some group training, where you live will determine how many choices you have. In a metro area, there may be a lot of options. In a rural area, it may be challenging to find a class that suits your needs.

When you are looking for a class, your first urge is to think about what you can't do. You think you can't dance or you haven't danced in years. Or maybe a class looks like fun, but you don't know if you can keep up. And what will people think if you can't do what's required. The only way to find out is to give it a try. Believe me, most people are busy trying to keep up in class. They are not watching you.

You are asking the wrong questions. First, let's assume you have the balance for the class. You don't have to be able to do every step or move to get started. You don't even need to finish the whole class. You need to do what you can. In other words, you just need to try.

I know from experience that worrying about looking silly, being slow, or not learning the moves fast enough are all concerns, but you can't let them stop you. You can't give up, and you can't stop. You don't have time. If classes are what you take, just make sure you can stay safe while you're doing them. If you need a chair class or a class with a chair to hold on to, find one. Find the right level for you. But don't give up because you think you're too old or too slow.

If you are going to work out at home, then you

can always start with bodyweight training. Starting with bodyweight training means you don't have to buy equipment to get started. You can find simple bodyweight workouts online. SilverSneakers and the organizations I've already mentioned will have bodyweight workouts.

If you have picked out a virtual program to follow, they will tell you what equipment you need. You will most likely need dumbbells; some use resistance bands, and some offer their proprietary equipment for sale, like unique barbells. You also may need a yoga mat to keep your feet from slipping if you are doing mobility or yoga. Most virtual training requires a subscription, but many provide lots of options for training. For virtual bodyweight programs, all you need is a computer screen or tablet to follow along. I find cell phone screens too small to see the workouts, but that's just me.

With your fitness program, you can mix and match. Remember Carol? She uses a virtual subscription service to supplement her classes and personal training. For Carol, variety is the spice of life. She always has a way to get her workouts in, even when she's not at the gym. Lynn supplements her workouts with biking, and Chuck plays tennis. I shouldn't say "supplements" because Chuck is improving his tennis game by doing resistance training. Lynn biked sixty-eight miles on her last birthday, and Carol took her kettlebell on a cross-country trip and took daily videos of her kettlebell workouts. They train to support all the other personal goals they have in their lives.

Now you've built out your schedule; it's time to set goals. What is it you want to accomplish? What is the one most important thing on your list? For many of my clients, it's leg strength. They want to get out of bed, off the couch, or easily out of a restaurant booth. They are beginning to feel frail, and they don't like it.

You may have a goal that is a combination of endurance and strength. You might want to be able to walk across a big box store without running out of energy. You might want to be able to climb the stairs at a friend's house so that you can visit them. You may want to take a walking tour of Europe. Your goals are your own. Write them down, work toward them, share them with your trainer if you have one. When you reach your goals, write down new ones. It's a never-ending process.

Measure where you are now so you can document your improvements. If you're working with a trainer, they may provide some tests that can be re-taken in a few months. If you are paying for training, you want to make sure you have a way to measure your progress.

Do not use the scale to measure your fitness progress. Muscle takes up less space than fat. I have clients who are losing inches but haven't lost a pound. You can measure your progress by how you feel, how your clothes fit, and whether you are reaching your goals. If you have been fighting the battle of the scale for most of your adult life, it's time to try a different approach.

Build some simple tests to track your progress. Again, your tests come from your goals. You might track how far or how many steps you can take now and test that again in six weeks. How many stairs can you climb with ease compared to how many you can climb in six weeks? If you're at a gym and can't think how to test your goal, ask the staff there. They should be able to help you decide on how to test for improvement. Revisit your goals. When you complete a goal, add a new one. Remember, if you're not moving forward, you're moving backward. Those are the only two choices we have.

Re-evaluate on a regular schedule. You should be sore after a good workout, but you shouldn't hurt so much you are incapacitated. DOMS, delayed onset muscle syndrome, is simply soreness after a workout. It's a good thing, and as your muscle repairs, you end up with more muscle. Building muscle is what you want to do. But if you are in such pain you don't ever want to work out again, rethink your workouts. Make them more manageable and work up to more difficulty.

If you measure your goals and find that you are making no progress, then re-evaluate your programming. Are you progressively increasing the weights you are using? If you are doing the exact time/weight/ distance twelve weeks from the day you started, you won't progress. You don't have to increase time/

distance/weight by a significant amount, but you have to increase it incrementally as you improve.

For example, if you can do a bicep curl with five pounds, increase the weight to eight pounds when it becomes easy. You may not be able to do as many curls with the eight pounds, but as you consistently train, that eight pounds will become easy.

If you look around, you might find something you love. You may be doing the resistance training because you have to, but you love your cardio classes. You might discover that you love feeling strong. I fell in love with kettlebells, and that love continues as I learn more skills. There are so many choices; don't be miserable doing something you hate. Look around for something you enjoy doing. If you are trying something new, give yourself enough time to decide if it's providing the benefits you want. If the answer is yes, maybe you tolerate the training but enjoy the gains you are making.

If you lifted weights as a young man, nothing stops you from working with weights again. You have to start light and move up, but there are no signs on the dumbbells or cables that say "young people only." It's hard, but if you can get past the thought that you're too old or don't belong, the gym can become a refuge.

You've met Lynn and Carol. They do both group and personal training. Neither were ready to attack the free weights alone, but we attack them together once a week. Carol is working on leg and glute strength, and Lynn is working on upper body strength. But I will let them tell their stories:

Carol: "Although I take group classes three days a week, I felt a personal trainer would help me build my confidence, make sure my form was good, and teach me how to use all the equipment. I was intimidated by the free weights and cables because I didn't know how to manipulate the weights and pick them up correctly. My trainer has helped me learn how to pick them up whether I am lying down, standing, squatting, or using a machine. Also, she has taught me when to ask for a spotter or lower the weight I am using. I maximize my time during personal training by doing exercises designed to meet my specific goals. My trainer knows my strengths and abilities, and she gives me her undivided attention. She pushes me to work harder than I would in a group class."

Lynn: "While the group sessions have helped me increase strength and endurance overall, I felt my upper body wasn't as strong as I wanted. Thus, I began personal training. While I'm developing weak areas, I am also mentally challenged as I learn to use different equipment and weights in alternate ways. As I'm learning how to use the equipment, I'm beginning to feel more confident in using the weight area on my own."

Carol talked about the functional benefits she has gained while Training to Age. Carol has seen outward changes, but she has also experienced better bone health and improved balance. She's also developed strength and energy and has more confidence in the gym. She said her favorite benefit is a community of positive, like-minded people. Even as active agers, there is nothing more fun than having someone else to play with.

Jan and John, two of my group clients, have also seen functional benefits. Jan can now reach up and take things off a shelf, and she noted that reaching up, in general, was easier. She's seen positive physical changes and laughs when she says she has a waist now. She can hold a plank, and although she has A-fib, she continues to build more stamina. John is working on stronger legs and more energy; he also continues to see results.

As I said in the beginning, you are training to live fully. Your goal is to enjoy all the things you have planned for your retirement for as long as possible.

Before we leave this chapter, we should probably touch on excuses. You will always have a reason to avoid working out. Every day is different. The main excuse is that you are just too "old" to start working out. I think I'll let two of my older clients respond to that one. I asked Jan and John if their age, seventy-six, provided a good reason not to work out. Jan quickly responded, "You are kidding me! You're never too old to start. There is always something you can do no matter what condition you are in. We are seventy-six. I don't know how you live independently if you're not working out."

John also had an opinion. "That's ridiculous. There is always something you can do. You have to keep moving. You have to be flexible, or you're not going to survive. I believe if you can't put your socks on, it's a short trip to needing care."

I have clients with many different medical conditions that range from diabetes to cancer. We all deal with bad knees, fussy shoulders, and body parts in general that don't work like they used to. I have clients who are cancer survivors and clients with pacemakers. Doing the work isn't easy for anyone. But I don't think I have a single client who won't tell you that doing the work is worth it.

You're retired, so more than likely, you can find thirty minutes six days a week. If you can't go to the gym, there are many virtual options. There will always be an excuse not to work out, but you only have this one life to live. Sometimes you just have to do the hard thing until it's not so hard anymore, or maybe use that twenty seconds of courage to get started.

If you want the benefits, you have to do the work. The rule is to progress slowly, steadily, and safely. Find something you genuinely enjoy doing, and it will change your life. I know most women of our generation don't have much experience with strength training. If you're thinking, *Not me, I'm sticking to the treadmill*, let me tell you in the next chapter why that's not an option.

CHAPTER 8

Just for Women

"If you think lifting is dangerous, try being
weak. Being weak is dangerous."

—Bret Contreras

YOU'VE JUST FINISHED all the preceding chapters,
and it sounds like a great idea except for one thing...
resistance training. If you are female and are comfortable with a dumbbell, kettlebell, or barbell, this chapter is not for you. However, if you're a woman who
finds anything but the treadmill or elliptical frightening, hang in here with me for a little bit longer.

Although girls today have many opportunities to
participate in sports at all ages and levels, most of our
generation didn't. We didn't have girls' sports at my
high school until 1974, a year after I graduated. You
will see young women today using all areas in the

gym. They are as comfortable using free weights as they are using the treadmill. I want you to be as comfortable as they are.

I joined gyms after I was married. I took aerobic classes, walked on the treadmill, climbed the stair climber, and that's about it. I used machines in the gym but never got comfortable with them. It never crossed my mind to pick up a dumbbell, learn to use a resistance band, or give the suspension training a try.

And when I did finally discover the barbell, it was forty-plus years after high school graduation. I still contend with friends telling me that deadlifting will make me look like a man. Or that I will get hurt because women shouldn't lift any more than ten pounds. That one cracks me up. We carry groceries and babies and kids, and of course, no one rips them out of our arms lest we get hurt. Pick up your forty-pound grandson; that's fine. If you pick up a forty-pound kettlebell, people stare in horror until they realize you know what you're doing. We haul vacuum cleaners and dirty clothes up and down stairs. And there is a fair chance that we will care for an ailing husband. It seems that people recognize that women need strength, but no one wants to watch them get strong.

My female clients in their sixties and seventies understand the importance of getting and staying strong enough to live a full and active life. I want you to know before you're seventy that staying strong is a lot easier than getting strong. Doing something new is hard. It's tough as we get older, and I realize I am asking you to step out of your comfort zone—way out of your comfort zone for some of you. But, if you've read the preceding chapters, you know what's at stake.

I am not willing to give up my ability to live independently. Given a choice of strength or frailty, I will choose strength. And I am betting you will too. I don't want to spend my last days lying in a nursing home with a broken hip. Let's be clear. I'm not saying I can avoid the misadventures of old age just by doing resistance training. But I can, most certainly, give myself the best chance possible. Resistance training is an essential part of healthy aging and not one I'm willing to give up.

I might know a little about you. If you've never stepped off the treadmill, now is the time to do it. I know it's a scary thought. And that's one of the reasons I am suggesting a trainer. For me, it was easy to work with machines, dumbbells, and even barbells, with my trainer providing direction.

Working out alone was hard for me in the beginning. I would worry that I'd do something wrong or use a dumbbell or barbell in a way that would make me look stupid. And I worried that people would laugh at an old lady trying to get strong so late in life. I worried about everything. It took me years to figure out that I was wasting energy on worry. A few people looked at me like I was a crazy lady, but most people either wished me good luck or asked me to show them how to do what I was doing. I almost passed out from fear the first time I competed in front of an audience. In reality, I received good wishes, high-fives, and a trophy. That's not what I expected.

Here's the first thing you need to know regardless of what type of resistance training you do. When you first step foot in a gym or a class, it feels like the whole world is watching, but, in truth, no one is. Or if they are, it's in wonder that you're willing to work out "at your age." Most people in a gym don't spend a lot of time worrying about what other people are doing. They are too busy doing their own thing.

Let's hear from Carol about her gym experience. "I was hopeful but cautious when I joined my gym at the age of sixty-one that I would feel comfortable and achieve my fitness goals. I am grateful to say that any concern I had went away almost immediately. It was a challenge, but I met my original goals and continue to achieve new ones. A lot of that success is due to the encouragement from what I like to refer to as my "gym family"; trainers and people I work out with who keep cheering me on!"

So, I hope I've convinced you to take that first step. You have to do bodyweight training or pick up that dumbbell, band, kettlebell, or barbell. You always start light and work your way up to a little more weight or a few more reps. If you want to learn to use a barbell, dumbbell, or kettlebell, find someone to teach you. If medicine balls or battle ropes look like fun, give them a try. The more equipment you learn how to use, the more engaging your gym experience will be.

If you need to, find a trainer or a class to help you get started. Give yourself a chance to get comfortable. Don't tell me old dogs can't learn new tricks. I know you can. You can learn to do resistance training with or without a trainer, and you can build strength. Remember that you can use your body weight as resistance, so strength training doesn't have to be complicated.

I talked about DOMS (delayed onset muscle syndrome) previously but wanted to mention it again. When you start working out, you may be sore. If you've never worked out, you may wonder if the pain indicates an injury. You may also wonder why you would want to go back and exercise again, only to be in pain the next day.

If it's just DOMS, the pain should be gone in a day or so. I'm fond of a hot shower, which always seems to help. Don't stop moving. Continuing to move is good for you and will help keep you from getting stiff. If you are in extreme pain, that is an entirely different discussion. See your doctor.

If you find DOMS unmanageable, dial back your workouts a bit and then slowly move forward. That might mean lowering the weight you're working with or reducing the time or repetitions. Just don't give up. I am usually sore after a workout but, for me, that little bit of pain means I'm taking my body forward, not backward. DOMS will be less impactful the longer you work out.

Let's talk a little about machines. Your urge will be to have someone show you how to use the line of machines in the gym. Machines are an excellent way to get started, but don't let them be the only tools you learn to use. There is a whole world of resistance training tools to explore. Use different tools to stay active and engaged. Variety is the spice of life!

Don't hesitate to ask for help. Most people will answer a question if you ask them, as will gym staff. You might avoid asking anyone with their hood up and their headphones on. That is usually the *leave me alone* signal. If you see someone working with a trainer, it's best not to interrupt. The trainer should be focusing on his client. The fear of asking is always much worse than the actual act of asking for help.

Here is something you may need to address. If you are at high risk for a fracture due to osteoporosis, you need to talk to your doctor and find out how to stay safe in the gym. You may need to work with a trainer. The point of going to the gym or taking a class is not to end up with a broken bone. That said, I have many people in my regular group classes with osteoporosis.

If you are working with a trainer in any setting, tell them that you have osteoporosis to help you train safely. Don't hide your medical issues. I work with all kinds of medical problems in both men and women. The only way a trainer can create an appropriate training program is to understand your medical history. You want programming designed for you. Or, when using a generic program or taking a class, ask for modifications if you need them.

A fitness professional who is aware of your medical history should be happy to help design appropriate programming specifically for you. You may have a knee replacement and find it difficult to kneel. Maybe the exercise can be modified to be done standing, seated, or using a pad for your knee. Range of motion can be an issue with shoulders, and your trainer can modify a pushup or press so that you can do it safely.

And this is where trust comes in. A trainer or group instructor will push you and ask you to challenge yourself. That's their job. Go up a little in weight. Do one more rep. You will be amazed at the results.

In my experience, women do very well in group classes. They enjoy the camaraderie of a group and are very good at supporting each other. If you can find suitable classes, not only will you learn to appreciate the workout, but you may make lifelong friends. And remember, whoever is leading your class should be able to modify the exercises if necessary. I often see women start a new group class believing they physically can't keep up, and they sail through the class with ease. Take a deep breath and have faith in yourself. Give a group class a try. You may be very pleasantly surprised by the outcome.

If you are working out at home, remember the

number one rule is to stay safe. Modify movements where you need to. There are many good choices for virtual training at home.

You can do this. Be brave and take each day one step at a time. Do the work and reap the benefits. Everything new is hard, but the rewards are going to be worth it.

Conclusion

"All stories have a beginning, a middle, and an ending, and if they're any good, the ending is a beginning."

—James Clavell

MANY OF US walk down the path to old age without learning all we can do to make the journey easier. If I've convinced you that you can positively impact your journey with exercise, I've done my job.

We've talked about aging and the myths surrounding aging and exercise. We've talked about the five dimensions of training, and I hope you understand the benefits of a combination program of resistance training, cardio, power, mobility, and stability—and all the different ways you can find programs that help you meet your goals.

If you are going to train, train for the results that will keep you strong and independent. Find a way to train that keeps you excited and engaged, because that engagement is your ticket to success. You don't have to love the process of building bone, muscle, power, endurance, and stability, but I hope you learn to love the results of all that work. Let those results drive you back to the gym or the class hungry for more.

You have many choices, including using trainers, taking classes, finding local and online active ager resources, or even working out at home. You can make your workouts even more fun by including friends and then going out for coffee afterward. And with planning your time, training can feel less like work and more like play!

The trip through old age isn't fun. Even in the best of cases, we're all approaching the end of the line. And the last few miles are going to be rough for most of us. But now, you have some tools that may make the ride less bumpy and a little easier to traverse. With work, you can make that period where your quality of life declines only a fraction of the last twenty or thirty years of your life.

Build a workout plan that works for you. If you're a woman who has never done resistance training, be brave and give it a try. There is nothing like feeling strong and moving well when you are sixty, seventy, or eighty. Remember, you have lots of options for training. If you want to stay engaged when you are doing your cardio, do what you enjoy. You can dance, walk, run, swim or play racquet sports. The list is endless.

For your mobility practice, you also have options. Some strength and aerobic classes will have mobility built-in. Yoga and tai chi help with mobility/flexibility, strength, and stability. Classes that target the active ager may have shoulder and hip mobility built-in.

Hate the thought of picking up a dumbbell? There are all kinds of tools, medicine balls, kettlebells, bands, barbells, even bodyweight. If you are moving against resistance, you are doing strength training. Hug a gallon of milk, stand up and sit down ten times and you're doing strength training.

There is no single path or tool that's right for everyone. Try lots of new classes and tools. You may be surprised by what you discover about yourself and your abilities. Listen to that voice in your head that suggests you should try something new because it looks interesting.

Turn off the voice that tells you you're too old and out of shape to try anything new. That voice is a liar.

So here are the rules:

#1 – Train at your level

Get clearance from your physician. Training is a marathon, not a sprint. Start slowly and work up to your goal of three hours per week. Stay safe and injury-free. Recovering from injuries can eat up a lot of time where you could be training.

#2 - Train three hours per week

> You can train in six sessions of thirty minutes, four sessions of forty-five minutes, or three one-hour sessions. You can mix it up, but you need to get your 180 minutes in each week. If you need to, start slowly and work up to three hours.

#3 - Train strength

> You can train strength in the gym, with a trainer, in a class, or virtually. There are many ways to train strength. You will need to find what works for you. Make sure your strength training includes building strong legs for stability. Strength training may also include single leg work and some speed work to increase your power.

#4 – Train cardio

> Pick one or two sessions to train cardio. One session could be long and slow cardio. One session could be endurance and speed. Use your imagination. You may already dance, play a racquet sport, take a step class or kickboxing class. There are many options. Find what works for you.

#5 – Train Mobility

> You may do your stretching and mobility work within your strength or cardio classes or find a yoga or tai chi class you love. Your goal is to make sure your training includes moving your joints through their full range of motion multiple times each week.

The dimensions you want to train—strength, power, endurance, stability, and mobility— will cross the boundaries of different types of training. Your job is to find three hours per week to get them all in. Training to Age is your new job, and it comes with many benefits. To reap these benefits, all you have to do is consistently invest three hours a week. "Consistently" is the most important word in this sentence. Think of this as your new part-time job that comes with lots of perks.

Now that you know you have some control over how you age, take the next steps. Set goals, create a schedule for your training, and make it a priority. The earlier you start, the better the outcome. Remember the term "compression of morbidity." Your goal is to compress the amount of time you are frail and dependent into as short a period as possible. You've earned this retirement; now live it as your best you!

References and Resources

Broadhouse, K. M., Singh, M. F., Sou, C., Gates, N., Wen, W., Brodaty, H., Jain, N., Wilson, G. C., Meiklejohn, J., Singh, N., Baune, B. T., Baker, M., Foroughi, N., Wang, Y., Kochan, N., Ashton, K., Brown, M., Li, Z., Mavros, Y., & Valenzuela, M. J. (2020). Hippocampal plasticity underpins long-term cognitive gains from resistance exercise in MCI. *NeuroImage: Clinical, 25*, 1-13. https://doi.org/10.1016/j.nicl.2020.102182

Cenidoza, D. (2015, April 30). *Strength after sixty—resilience against frailty: Part 1.* Strong Medicine. https://strongmedicine.dragondoor.com/strength-after-sixty-resilience-against-frailty-part-i/

Dominic, A. (2019, September 3). *Seniors can effectively build muscle regardless of previous habits, new study finds.* Club Industry. https://www.clubindustry.com/fitness-studies/seniors-can-effectively-build-muscle-regardless-previous-habits-new-study-says

Harvard Health Publishing. (2016, February 19). *Declining muscle mass is part of aging, but that does not mean you are helpless to stop it.* https://www.health.harvard.edu/staying-healthy/preserve-your-muscle-mass

Jo, S. (2014, November 15). *Balance training for the glutes and abs.* Ace. https://www.acefitness.org/education-and-resources/professional/expert-articles/5166/balance-training-for-the-glutes-and-abs/

Joshua, A. M., D'Souza, V., Unnikrishnan, B., Mithra, P., Kamath, A., Acharya, V., & Venugopal, A. (2014). Effectiveness of progressive resistance strength training versus traditional balance exercise in improving balance among the elderly—a randomized controlled trial. *Journal of Clinical and Diagnostic Research, 8*(3), 98-102. https://doi.org/10.7860/jcdr/2014/8217.4119

Latona, V. (2019, May 15). *How to find time for exercise.* AARP. https://www.aarp.org/health/healthy-living/info-2019/committing-to-exercise.html

Lawrence, B. (2015). Training the brain to change the way we age, part 1: Understanding neuroplasticity. *The Journal on Active Aging, 14*(2), 36-42. https://www.findlawrence.com/articles/Article-JAA-Training-the-brain-pt1.pdf

Levine, H. (2019, June 12). *Strength training's surprising health benefits.* AARP. https://www.aarp.org/health/healthy-living/info-2019/strength-training-health-benefits.html

Liu, Y., Lee, D. C., Li, Y., Zhu, W., Zhang, R., Sui, X., Lavie, C. J., Blair, S. N. (2018). Associations of resistance exercise with cardiovascular disease morbidity and mortality. *Medicine & Science in Sports & Exercise, 51*(3), 499-508. http://doi. org/100.1249/MSS.0000000000001822

Neighmond, P. (2011, February 21). *Seniors can still bulk up on muscle by pressing iron.* NPR. https://www.npr.org/2011/02/21/133776800/ seniors-can-still-bulk-up-on-muscle-by-press- ing-iron

Olds, J. (2014, December 14). *Age is no barrier to lifting heavy objects.* stuff. https://www.stuff. co.nz/life-style/well-good/inspire-me/64055515/

Phillips Smith, M., Müller, Neidenbach, R., Ewert, P., & Hager, A. (2018, November 16-17). *Handgrip strength is associated with lung function, but not oxygen uptake, in several congenital heart defects across the lifespan.* American College of Cardiology Latin America Conference. Lima, Peru. https://www.research- gate.net/publication/329010345

Puszczalowska-Lizis, E., Bujas, P., Jandzis, S., Omorczyk, J., & Zak, M. Inter-gender differ- ences of balance indicators in persons 60-90 years of age. *Clinical Interventions in Aging, 13*, 903-912. https://doi.org/10.2147/cia.s157182

Reiner, V. (2020, February 11). *Strength training can help protect the brain from degeneration.* The University of Sydney. https://www.sydney.

edu.au/news-opinion/news/2020/02/11/strength-training-can-help-protect-the-brain-from-degeneration.html

Rizzo, N. (2021, May 21). *78 science-backed benefits of weightlifting for seniors*. RunRepeat. https://runrepeat.com/weightlifting-benefits-seniors

Skelton, D. (2015, October 8). *Explainer: Why does our balance get worse as we grow older?* The Conversation. https://theconversation.com/explainer-why-does-our-balance-get-worse-as-we-grow-older-48197

Weiner, Z. (2021, June 18). *I'm a cardiologist, and these are the 5 best strength-training moves for boosting your heart health*. Well & Good. https://www.wellandgood.com/is-strength-training-good-for-your-heart/